Governors State University
Library
Hours:
Monday thru Thursday 8:30 to 10:30
Friday and Saturday 8:30 to 5:00
Sunday 1:00 to 5:00 (Fall and Winter Trimester Only)

DEMCO

DEFYING DEMENTIA

Understanding and Preventing Alzheimer's and Related Disorders

Robert Levine, MD

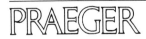

Westport, Connecticut
London

Library of Congress Cataloging-in-Publication Data

Levine, Robert, 1939–
    Defying dementia : understanding and preventing Alzheimer's and
related disorders / Robert Levine.
        p. cm.
    Includes bibliographical references and index.
    ISBN 0–275–98970–4 (alk. paper)
    1. Dementia. I. Title.
    RC521.L48   2006
    616.8'3—dc22   2006008236

British Library Cataloguing in Publication Data is available.

Library of Congress Catalog Card Number: 2006008236
ISBN: 0–275–98970–4

First published in 2006

Praeger Publishers, 88 Post Road West, Westport, CT 06881
An imprint of Greenwood Publishing Group, Inc.
www.praeger.com

Printed in the United States of America

The paper used in this book complies with the
Permanent Paper Standard issued by the National
Information Standards Organization (Z39.48–1984).

10 9 8 7 6 5 4 3 2 1

To my mother Dorothy
    who was always so alive and now lingers with dementia,
And to my patients with dementia and their families,
    from whom I have learned so much.

CONTENTS

PREFACE

If I had known
That old age would call,
I'd have shut my gate,
Replied 'Not at home!'
And refused to meet him.

Anonymous Poem from *Kokinshu*[1]

"A physician cannot improve on an asymptomatic patient!" This was a favorite aphorism of a professor of mine during my training in neurology decades ago. He was trying to convey the idea to his resident physicians that when people feel well, you don't make them feel better by treating them. And since they won't see any benefits from your treatment, it won't make them happier. In fact, they may be unhappier because of restrictions you try to impose, or medications you want them to take.

My professor's admonition is a significant part of the dilemma we face in dealing with dementia. How do we induce people to address a potential problem on the distant horizon when they currently feel well? How do we motivate individuals to take action, or change behavior, in response to a possible threat that has not yet materialized? It is an issue of considerable importance because the earlier the campaign is initiated to defeat this unseen foe, the greater the chances the combatant will emerge victorious. This dilemma is a challenge for physicians who specialize in cognitive problems. Strategies for preventing dementia are most effective if they are started while we are young, before intellectual decline has begun. I am not proposing that we all embark on an outlandish prescription of boring mental exercises and special diets, along with a shopping list of various substances we must ingest in order to enhance memory and thinking. Instead, I am suggesting some simple actions that should be embedded in a healthy lifestyle to protect our minds and bodies: mostly common sense.

This book is meant to serve both as a guide and as a reference to understanding and preventing dementia. It is presented in two parts. Before we consider the necessary steps to prevent dementia, we should know what it is and understand it in all its forms. There may be some slogging through the technical passages, particularly in the first part, but some of the science can be skimmed if it is too difficult or not of interest. It is more important to have a general overview of the various types of dementia and see how these processes cause us to lose our minds. There is a glossary that explains many of the scientific terms and will help to decipher any perplexing statements. The second part that focuses on prevention is easier to grasp and provides most of the meat (or in this case fish) for the necessary meal.

We do have some control over this destructive force called dementia, and with proper actions on our part we can achieve mastery. But it may require a certain degree of discipline and perhaps abandoning some ingrained habits. The transformation may not be easy. But recognizing the scourge that dementia is, and the way it devours the humanity of its victims, may inspire us to move ahead. Preparation is the key word in combating this adversary: building solid defenses over time. And while any moment is worthwhile to begin this task, the earlier the better.

This book is intended for intelligent lay people interested in learning about dementia and the measures that can be taken to repel its onslaught. It should also be of interest to caregivers and family members of impaired patients. Those health professionals in the trenches who deal with dementia first hand and want to decipher what is happening to their charges, may find it helpful as well. (The case histories used are disguised to protect the identity of the patients.)

ACKNOWLEDGEMENTS

I would like to thank Randi and Shelly Frank, Steve and Avor Breiner and Joyce Hobbie for their review of the manuscript, criticism and suggestions which were very helpful. My son Matthew Levine also provided comments and ideas that were valuable in shaping the book. Dr. Sam Markind added his professional scrutiny from a neurological standpoint. Dr. Barney Frank, a gegriatrician, was sharp-eyed and critical, his assistance and advice particularly beneficial.

The Norwalk Hospital librarian, Ms. Jill Golrick, aided me with my research and the Westport Library librarian, Ms. Margie Den, offered some practical ideas.

I am also grateful to my editor at Greenwood Press, Debora Carvalko, who helped to get this project off the ground and see it through to fruition.

My wife Anne, as always, was a source of encouragement and love, but also someone I could bounce my ideas off of while I was working and get thoughtful feedback. Her reading of the manuscript also resulted in astute comments which aided in the development of the book. She is indeed an incredible muse.

Robert A. Levine
Westport, CT
March 25, 2006

Part I

UNDERSTANDING DEMENTIA

Chapter 1

INTRODUCTION

Youth is a gift of nature; aging is a work of art.

Anonymous

Bill, an 83-year-old former salesman in good physical health, lived with his 78-year-old wife, Loretta, in a small Connecticut city. His wife had heart disease which limited her activities. They had two sons on the West Coast who saw them infrequently. Most of their friends had moved away. One day, Loretta sent her husband to the local pharmacy, a quarter of a mile away, to pick up a renewal of her heart medication. Bill left the house at about 3:10 in the afternoon. When he had not returned by 5:30, his wife informed the police who searched the entire city and neighboring towns, but there was no sign of him or the car. The following day, police units throughout the state and most of the East Coast were notified to look out for him. The sons flew back to Connecticut to be with their mother. On the third day, Bill was finally located in Brooklyn. His car had run out of gas and was stalled in the middle of the road. When the city police came, they found a confused old man who had no idea where he was or how he had gotten there. Though he still had his credit cards and license, there was no money in his wallet. His sons came to retrieve him, and took him and the car back home.

Teresa was a divorced 59-year-old woman who lived alone in a tiny house in a shoreline town. Employed after her divorce as a teacher's aide, she had stopped working 10 years earlier. She had one daughter, a single mother with two young children, who had a full time job and visited only on the holidays. Teresa had been smoking one to two packs of cigarettes since she was a teenager, and was also known to drink heavily when she went out with friends, two women about her age whom she saw intermittently. Three months earlier, on the July 4th weekend, one of the neighbors had commented to the daughter that her mother wasn't keeping up the house, with weeds overgrown and paint peeling from the siding. When the daughter spoke to Teresa, she said she would handle it. Eventually, Teresa was brought by her daughter for a neurologic consultation because her speech was not making sense at times and she had neglected to pay her bills.

Renee, a retired interior decorator, was brought into the hospital one evening with congestive heart failure and was found to be disoriented. A 77-year-old woman, she lived with her 89-year-old husband, Clark, who had been disabled by a stroke. They had a townhouse in a condominium complex in an affluent town. Childless, they had been married for over 50 years. Round the clock health aides cared for her husband. In the hospital ICU, blood tests revealed that Renee's digoxin level (a medication used to regulate heart activity) was very low. It was discovered after considerable probing that she had stopped taking her medications about a week earlier. When questioned why, she was reluctant to answer at first, but then told her physician that one of the female aides had been trying to poison her with those pills. Though she was confused and her story was not coherent, she insisted that this aide was in love with Clark and trying to steal him.

Jack had been a teacher and his wife, Thelma, an administrator in the local school system and they occupied a comfortable apartment in a medium-sized city. They had two married children living several hundred miles away, whom they saw rarely. Now 68, Jack had been retired for 5 years. With no special interests, he watched television most days, occasionally going out for dinner with Thelma. About two years earlier, his personality had seemed to change. He had always been outgoing, but then began constantly cracking jokes, many of them off color, and making inappropriate comments to acquaintances, embarrassing Thelma and their friends. He would also get into arguments at times over unimportant matters. Eventually, their friends refused to socialize with them, and family members stopped visiting. Jack became increasingly disorganized as well, missing appointments and delaying payment of bills. At her insistence, he went to see a physician and was referred to a psychiatrist, who then sent him to a neurologist. On testing, he was fully oriented with intact recall and memory, and calculated and reasoned fairly well. But he quipped throughout the interview and examination, making comments at times that were rude and disrespectful.

Louis was a 68-year-old man whose wife had died of cancer about 10 years earlier. He was estranged from his only son and lived by himself in a small cottage in a working-class neighborhood of a city on the coast. A former deliveryman for an oil company, he had not worked for five years and was known in the area as a recluse. About twice a week, he drove to the store to pick up groceries, unloading them, then retreating into his house. Occasionally, he would be out mowing the lawn, though that activity had stopped six months before. Unless addressed directly, he rarely said a word to the neighbors, but seemed friendly enough if he was asked a question. One cold, gray afternoon in November, he was seen walking down the street barefoot in an open bathrobe. When the woman next door ran after him, he did not seem to know who she was and was not clear about where he was going. The police brought him to the hospital where he was admitted for evaluation.

Bob was a retired executive who with his wife, Jackie, resided in a lovely home on the river in a small inland town. They had three married children in nearby communities with seven grandchildren. Bob was an avid golfer, loved to play bridge with his wife and enjoyed dining out. About six months earlier, his family noted that his walking had changed. He seemed to be taking smaller steps and shuffling at times. Shortly afterward, he began to have occasional urinary incontinence and his memory wasn't quite as good as it had been. Though his family urged him to see a doctor, he resisted for a while. He finally agreed after acknowledging that his walking was impaired.

The individuals described above have been attacked by dementia. It did not arise overnight in any of them, but was a slow, relentless process that affected their brains and robbed them of normal acuity and cognitive function over time. Dementia was not diagnosed earlier because they lived alone or with companions who were not perceptive enough to realize that a serious problem existed. Sometimes denial by the family, or the affected person, may also prevent a diagnosis from being made until the abnormalities are so obvious, they cannot be explained away by rationalizations or excuses.

The possibility of developing dementia terrifies many people as they grow older, recognizing that their mental faculties may deteriorate and they can be left as empty shells of their former selves, incapable of managing their lives. It is particularly frightening for those who have seen family members or friends afflicted by this scourge, with loss of memory and the ability to think. Though the risk is real for all of us, increasing as we age, and there is no absolute way to prevent dementia, there are numerous steps we can take to significantly lower the risk, enabling us to maintain our independence and quality of life. This book will describe the effects of normal aging on brain function and what is called mild cognitive impairment, as well as the various forms of dementia. It will then detail what we can do to keep our heads above the water and reduce the likelihood of our succumbing to the "dementing" process.

Dementia is not a disease. It is a condition caused by a number of different diseases. Many people equate dementia with Alzheimer's disease, but they are not synonymous though Alzheimer's is one of dementia's major causes. Dementia is a global impairment of cognitive ability that interferes with normal activities and everyday living, particularly involving a person's memory and executive function (planning and organization). What was once called senility is really dementia. It is not a normal part of aging though the diseases that produce it are much more common in the elderly. Because of this, the number of patients with dementia can be expected to rise dramatically in the years ahead as our population ages further. Dementia is a chronic condition that must be differentiated from delirium which occurs acutely, and also from depression. It is believed by many investigators that most degenerative diseases of the brain that cause dementia are the result of structural changes in brain proteins, with misfolding and abnormal aggregation of these substances.

DEMOGRAPHICS OF DEMENTIA

Until the last half of the twentieth century, dementia was relatively infrequent, as few individuals survived into what we would now consider old age. During most of recorded history, the average life expectancy was about 30 years, with infectious diseases, famine and wars placing a cap on population growth. By 1900, however, life expectancy had increased to about 50, mainly because of improved sanitation and agricultural production. At the start of the current millennium, most people in the Western world live into their late seventies or eighties, with many surviving into their nineties or even longer. Accompanying this extended survival, cases of dementia have been rising. And during the next century, as life expectancy continues to increase, one can anticipate an even greater explosion in the number of people with dementia, unless, of course, medical science finds effective ways to intervene.

About 12 percent of our population is now 65 or over, with about 5.5 percent 75 or above.[1] This is expected to grow to about 14.5 percent and 6 percent respectively as more baby boomers reach 65 in 2015. As they move into their seventies and eighties, more than 20 percent of our citizenry will be 65 or over, with 9 percent 75 or over. Currently, it is estimated that more than 4 million, to as many as 7 million, people in the United States have dementia and that more than 14 million people will be demented by the year 2050. At present, 5 to 10 percent of those 65 and older are believed to be demented, and 40 to 50 percent of those 85 and older. One report noted that "the prevalence and incidence of dementia doubles every five years in individuals between the ages of 65 and 95."[2] Of those who survive to age 100, 75 percent will be demented. Given these statistics, it is a frightening specter indeed for an aging population.

Dementia imposes a huge burden on both society and individuals. The economic costs are staggering and believed to be well over $100 billion annually at this time. Included in this are the expenses of treating the various forms of dementia, diagnostic tests and medication, home health care, part-time and full-time aides, nursing homes, etc. (Interestingly, only 3 out of 10 patients with dementia have ever received any treatment.) There is also the loss of productivity from those who have dementia, and diminished productivity from the family members who have assumed the responsibility for care.

The social and emotional costs are also immense. Dementia is extremely disruptive to family relationships, with the normal roles of parent and child often reversed. Children may have to look after parents whose cognitive function and behavior has regressed, and who are unable to care for themselves. This may start with managing the checkbook and finances of a mother or father who can't seem to keep the numbers straight. Sons and daughters may then have to take away driving privileges from parents or restrict other activities, even prohibiting them from leaving their homes without accompaniment. They may impose strangers upon them as caregivers, or force them to reside in nursing homes. Previous boundaries may be breached by children who have to clean up parents unable to control their bowels or bladders. And as many couples currently choose to have children later in life, they may find themselves caring for children as well as parents, the so-called sandwich generation.

CAUSES OF DEMENTIA

The statistics for the causes of dementia (Table 1.1) vary depending on the population surveyed and the criteria used for diagnosis of the different types. At times, causes may not be clear cut, and in many cases more than one pathologic process may be at work, so at best the statistics given are estimates. It is also true that the prevalence of the different forms varies in

Table 1.1
Common Causes of Dementia

Alzheimer's disease—50–75% of all dementia
Fronto-Temporal dementia (Pick's disease)—5–10%
Dementia with Lewy bodies and Parkinson's disease dementia—15–20%
Vascular dementia—20–25%
Mixed dementia—20–30%
(More than 100% because of overlap)

Table 1.2
Dementia in Great Britain

Alzheimer's disease—55%
Vascular dementia—20%
Dementia with Lewy Bodies—15%
Fronto-temporal dementia—5%
Other dementias—5%

different countries, and dementia seems to occur more frequently in urban environments than in rural areas.

The way the Alzheimer's Society in Great Britain breaks down the causes of dementia is noted in Table 1.2.

Mixed dementia is defined as a loss of cognitive ability due to two or more diseases affecting the brain simultaneously. Most commonly, this is Alzheimer's and multi-infarct disease (vascular dementia) seen together. But the combination of Alzheimer's and Dementia with Lewy bodies also occurs frequently. A less common cause of dementia, normal pressure hydrocephalus, may be present with Alzheimer's changes, vascular dementia, or both.

Overall, it is felt that Alzheimer's pathology is present in about two-thirds of all dementias, with the incidence in studies ranging from 42–81 percent.[3] A report from Italy in 2005 found Alzheimer's as the cause in 62.6 percent and vascular dementia in 29.6 percent.[4] Another larger study from countries throughout Europe had Alzheimer's in 53.7 percent (range 38.5–78 percent) and vascular dementia in 15.8 percent.[5] In countries where severe atherosclerosis and high blood pressure are pervasive, vascular dementia may be as prevalent, or even more prevalent than Alzheimer's disease. And sophisticated evaluation of patients may not be available in some areas, eliminating major subtypes of dementia in the statistics reported. Aside from the more common causes which will be discussed in subsequent chapters, there are various other conditions that can produce dementia which will also be addressed.

GENERAL CHARACTERISTICS OF DEMENTIA

There are certain characteristics common to the diverse forms of dementia, with particular features dominant in specific types. But even the same kind of dementia may appear in different ways, assume different shapes and run a variable course.

Loss of Memory

Loss of memory is the hallmark of dementia. It may not be the initial symptom in all cases, but generally occurs early in the course of the illness and at some point is found in everyone who is afflicted. Episodic (short-term) memory is usually involved, but eventually all types of memory fall prey to whatever destructive process is attacking the brain. In time, there is no recall of the important facts of our lives, or even recognition of those most dear to us. Our minds become blank slates, with a lifetime of learning and experience erased, and no new information able to be imprinted, or retained.

Since diminished memory plays such a conspicuous role in all forms of dementia, it is important that we understand something about it. Three steps are involved in the process of what we call memory. The first is the acquisition of information through our sensory systems, mainly vision and hearing, though the others (smell, taste and touch) are utilized as well. The second is the storage of the data obtained in some area or areas of our brains. The third step is the retrieval of information so that it can be used in some way, perhaps causing us to act, perhaps influencing our mood, perhaps unearthing other memories. A small structure called the hippocampus (a grouping of cells in the middle temporal lobe) is the part of the brain that sort of acts as a traffic cop for information, deciding what we will be able to access on a short-term basis, and what will be sent on to the cerebral cortex (the mantle of cells covering the cerebral hemispheres) for storage as long-term memory.

In the past, one spoke merely of short-term and long-term memory in describing how the brain worked. Short-term memory was impaired earlier and more severely in most dementias and injuries to the brain.

While this remains true to some degree, the story is much more complicated than that. Intact memory requires a number of systems within the brain operating together. "Four memory systems are of clinical relevance: episodic memory, semantic memory, procedural memory and working memory ... Different memory systems depend on different neuroanatomical structures. Some systems are associated with conscious awareness (explicit) and can be consciously recalled (declarative), whereas others are expressed by a change in behavior (implicit) and are typically unconscious (nondeclarative). ... A memory system is a way for the brain to process information that will be available for use at a later time."[6]

Episodic memory includes much of what we used to call short-term memory, though some of the knowledge may be retained for years. It is used to recall information from our daily lives, such as what we had for breakfast this morning, or an article in the newspaper. Though episodic memory is dependant on the integrity of the hippocampus and the medial (middle) temporal lobes, a number of other areas of the brain are also necessary. If this system is damaged or dysfunctional, there is difficulty learning new information and a problem retrieving information recently learned. Knowledge acquired in the more distant past usually remains intact. In addition to dementia, episodic memory can be impaired by injuries to the brain, a lack of oxygen, strokes, encephalitis (a viral infection of the brain) and multiple sclerosis. Temporary loss can occur after cerebral concussions, seizures or a poorly understood entity called transient global amnesia.

Semantic memory encompasses our overall body of facts and information, not derived from any particular memory, such as who wrote the Declaration of Independence, the size and color of an elephant, the most populous country in the world or the difference between a rake and a shovel. Though some investigators believe that semantic memory is stored in various areas of the cerebral cortex, it appears to be most affected by conditions that damage the inferolateral temporal lobes, particularly Alzheimer's disease. Deterioration of semantic memory appears to occur independently of episodic memory, suggesting that there are two distinct systems involved, though they both may be undermined by many of the same processes. Tests for the loss of semantic memory focus on having the person name familiar objects, and also describing items whose names he or she has been given.

Procedural memory involves learning and retaining certain skills that are utilized for the most part unconsciously and automatically, such as the use of a computer keyboard or mouse, or playing a musical instrument.

The parts of the brain activated by this type of memory include the supplementary motor area of the cortex (in the frontal lobes), the cerebellum (at the back of the brain) and the basal ganglia (deep in the cerebral hemispheres). Alzheimer's usually does not affect this type of memory until late in the course of the disease. Disorders that target the basal ganglia such as Parkinson's disease and Huntington's disease can degrade procedural memory, as can strokes involving the above structures.

Working memory requires keeping information available on a temporary basis to allow us to perform specific tasks, such as calling someone on the phone, or remembering how to drive to someone's home. Intact attention, concentration and short-term memory are necessary for working memory. Multiple areas of the cerebral cortex and subcortical areas may be utilized in this process, but the prefrontal cortex (frontal lobes) is most important. Diseases that cause extensive damage throughout the brain, particularly involving the frontal lobe and its connections, can produce a decline in working memory. This includes Alzheimer's disease, Huntington's, Parkinson's disease and dementia with Lewy bodies, as well as cerebrovascular disease, head trauma and multiple sclerosis.

It is important to remember that one disease process can affect several types of memory, presenting a picture that is not clear cut. Often in describing a person with memory problems, using short-term or long-term loss, or a combination of both, may be adequate.

Impaired Executive Function

This is another prime characteristic of dementia. By this is meant the inability to plan or organize one's life, then act upon the ideas that have been generated. There is difficulty with abstract reasoning and decision-making, a lack of any initiative and a passivity in dealing with unfamiliar situations. A failure to sustain goal directed behavior occurs and the person may act only on immediate concrete objectives. Executive function is a very important brain process that allows us to run our lives independently. Losing this ability can be quite disabling, even if memory is relatively intact. Problems with executive function are believed to result from damage to the frontal lobes. It is seen in all types of dementia, but earlier in the course of fronto-temporal dementia and Alzheimer's disease.

Language Function

Language function is also subverted in most cases of dementia. The difficulty can range from subtle changes in the use of words to total gibberish or even muteness when the disease process is advanced. Often the struggle to express oneself is more pronounced than understanding speech, but in time both aspects of language are compromised. There may be difficulty naming objects and the normal syntax of speech may be disrupted. This disintegration of language function is called aphasia and may be manifest in a number of ways, depending on the relative involvement of different areas of the brain.

An additional symptom in dementia is the inability to perform complex motor tasks though muscle strength may be intact. This is believed to occur because of a deficit of conceptualization of what an act entails and is defined as an apraxia. Though language function may seem normal with this, some degree of impairment is often associated.

Also noted occasionally in dementia can be a failure to recognize people, objects or even body parts, and an inability to comprehend their significance, even though the primary sense organs remain intact. The general term for this conundrum is agnosia.

Changes in Behavior

Changes in behavior are a frequent aspect of dementia and a cause of great concern for spouses and families. These include depression or apathy, agitation, paranoia and what can be called "disinhibition." This last term is used to describe the loss of the normal social restraints that guide our actions and are essential to relationships. (I have also seen disinhibition to a minor degree in normal aging and mild cognitive impairment.) The veil of politeness and courtesy that cloaks our behavior may be torn away by the disease process. Comments can be made that are insulting or hurtful to someone, without the speaker realizing the consequences of what he or she has said. In addition to verbal abuse, behavior can be seen that varies from rude or inappropriate conduct to dangerous acts. Inappropriate sexual advances to adults or even children may also occur occasionally.

Agitation is noted as well in many individuals with dementia at any stage of their illness. It may arise from intrinsic anxiety, perhaps as part of the disease, or may be due to constant unfamiliarity with that person's circumstances: not knowing where he or she is, how he or she got there, and what he or she is supposed to be doing. There is a disconnect from the surrounding world because of memory impairment and inability to reason, leading to anxiety and agitation. Paranoia also develops at times, perhaps related to similar factors. A wife may leave the house to go shopping and her husband can't remember where she's gone or when she's supposed to come back, so he starts believing she's having an affair with someone. Or an individual misplaces things in the house and thinks people are stealing from him.

One sad example of paranoid thinking involved an 88-year-old patient of mine with Alzheimer's disease. His wife was 85 and in a wheelchair after having been felled by a stroke. The patient believed his wife was having an affair with their 90-year-old neighbor who had been a friend of theirs for years. Using logic to show him the improbability of his notion was fruitless and he insisted the affair was taking place. Perhaps there had been some precipitating event, or he had fantasized about this in the past, or the idea has just arisen in his dysfunctional brain.

Depression and apathy are also common in dementia and may precede the clinical presentation in many cases, though it is currently unclear whether this is actually a manifestation of the disease process itself. (Depression is also felt to be a risk factor for the development of dementia.) It often occurs early in the course and may be due to some inherent mechanism. Another possibility is that the person with insipient dementia is aware at some level that he or she is losing cognitive ability and becomes depressed because of this. At times, it may be difficult to ascertain whether the dementia or depression is the primary process, and whether someone is presenting with a so-called pseudo-dementia. (This will be discussed later.)

Spatial Orientation

Spatial orientation is often impaired as well in individuals with dementia. This may result in people getting lost driving. Later on, they may lose their way walking in the neighborhood if they leave their homes unattended. As the disease progresses, they may even get lost within their homes, not knowing where various rooms are located. Memory dysfunction may play a role in addition to spatial relationships. The spatial problems may be seen if a person is asked to draw a clock with a particular time, or asked to draw or copy geometrical figures.

RISK FACTORS FOR DEMENTIA

If a small number of the brain's vast array of neurons (nerve cells) are damaged or destroyed, there may be no evidence of cognitive decline, or it may be very subtle and not interfere with a person's life. However, as more neurons are lost, problems with thinking begin to arise. Mild cognitive impairment may occur, leading finally to dementia. We should keep in mind that most investigators believe the changes in the brain that are responsible for dementia begin many years or even decades prior to the onset of symptoms. The most important risk factors are those that predispose us to the development of atherosclerosis, heart disease and strokes. Since a considerable percentage of cases of dementia result from cerebrovascular disease, or a combination of Alzheimer's with cerebrovascular disease, one would expect any factor favoring athero-sclerotic changes in the blood vessels to increase the incidence of dementia. Small vessel disease in the brain, and major or minor strokes, may cumulatively damage enough neurons to produce vascular dementia. Or enough neurons may be damaged to allow the underlying changes of Alzheimer's disease that had been slowly devouring the brain to finally emerge in a clinically apparent dementia. A number of articles in the medical literature have shown that small lesions in the white matter of the brain in older people correlate with a greater incidence of dementia.[7] It is believed that these are caused by tortuosity and atherosclerotic changes in the long penetrating arterioles (small arteries) that supply the white matter, making them vulnerable to any drop in blood flow in these vessels.

One large study evaluated a group of patients (8,845) medically from 1964 to 1973, when they were between the ages of 40 and 44.[8] Thirty years later, 721 of them, or 8.2 percent, had developed dementia. Smoking, hypertension, elevated cholesterol and diabetes at midlife were each found to have increased the risk of dementia in these people by 20–40 percent. The risk was doubled in those who had all four factors compared to those with none. Another report also indicated that diabetes heightened the possibility of developing Alzheimer's disease and cogni-tive decline.[9] Even prediabetes and insulin resistance makes dementia more likely. And midlife obesity has also been shown to significantly increase the chances of Alzheimer's disease and dementia later on.[10] Other vascular risk factors, such as elevated plasma homocysteine, C-reactive protein (CRP), interleukin 6, alpha 1-antichymotrysin levels all were associated with increased odds of developing dementia.[11] Simi-larly, the risk of dementia, both Alzheimer's and the vascular type, was amplified by elevated cholesterol and lipid levels in the blood.[12] Period-ontal disease was also found to be associated with a higher incidence of dementia, possibly because of the chronic infection and inflammation. Of course, all of these studies suggest possible avenues to reduce the risk. Again it should be emphasized that the prevalence of these various risk factors in midlife increased the chances of developing dementia later on, which means that preventive measures should be started early to obtain maximum benefit.

The APOE gene is a major determinant of risk for Alzheimer's disease, with carriers of APOE 4 having a significantly greater chance of getting Alzheimer's and getting it at an earlier age than noncarriers.[13] Even without dementia, they show more evidence of cognitive decline in middle age and have poorer outcomes after head injuries.[14] Those who are homozygous (have two copies of the gene, one from each parent) for APOE 4 are at more risk than those who are heterozygous (one copy). However, APOE 4 is not an absolute predictor of Alzheimer's and a large percentage of people with the gene do not get the disease. On the other hand, the APOE 2 gene appears to offer some protection against cognitive loss and dementia, as does APOE 3. Though APOE 4 carriers have higher levels of LDL and total cholesterol, and APOE 2 carriers have lower levels, the exact manner in which these genes influence the development of Alzheimer's disease and cognitive dysfunction is speculative.

A number of other individual risk factors of uncertain mechanism also seem to increase the possibility of dementia. As mentioned, depression, even in the distant past, heightens the risk. Head injuries make a person more susceptible. Low bone mineral density in older women appears to be associated with an increased chance of developing Alzheimer's and all types of dementia.[15] Reduced thyroid stimulating hormone may also be an independent risk factor for Alzheimer's[16] though it is not yet clear whether this finding precedes or follows the onset of the disease. Weight loss may be a predictor of dementia in older people (even though midlife obesity greatly increases its possibility), and may begin several years before cognitive decline is evident.[17] However, it is likely that the dementing process was already at work while the weight was being shed and the person may have been in the early or preclinical stages of dementia. Chronic stress over years or decades is believed to raise the risk, as does a family history of first degree relatives with dementia. And low educational status and jobs of low complexity make dementia more likely as well.

DIAGNOSING DEMENTIA

When a patient enters a doctor's office complaining of difficulty with memory or thinking, there are three questions the physician must answer. Is the patient truly demented? If so, what is the cause? Is there some process that is potentially reversible or can be arrested?

Table 1.3
Criteria for the Diagnosis of Dementia

Loss of memory and one or more other cognitive abilities (aphasia, apraxia,
   agnosia or disturbance in executive functioning)
Substantial impairment in social or occupational functioning (decline from a
   previous level of functioning)
Deficits that do not occur exclusively during the course of delirium[a]

---

[a]Claudia Kawas, "Early Alzheimer's Disease," *N Eng J Med*, 2003, 349: 1056–1063.

I have found as a rule of thumb that when someone is concerned about
memory loss but is unaccompanied by family members when visiting my
office, dementia is unlikely. A young person alone worried about his or
her memory is usually anxious or depressed. An older person with
memory problems may still be anxious or depressed, but may also
have age-related forgetfulness, or mild cognitive impairment. People
with dementia generally do not have enough insight into their problems
to seek medical help. It is usually family or friends who insist that a
physician be seen when memory is failing and the question of dementia
arises. Unfortunately, this often occurs rather late in the course of the
disease. Over 90 percent of early dementia is believed to go unrecognized
by family and friends, and as much as 50 percent of moderate dementia.
The criteria for the diagnosis of dementia is shown in Table 1.3.

All patients with the possibility of dementia require a hierarchy of
medical studies, though frequently a physician can decide whether the
condition is present merely by taking a history from the patient and
family. Decoding the type of dementia is more complicated since there
may be a considerable overlap in symptoms. A physical examination and
blood tests may be helpful in excluding medical causes, including B12
deficiency, thyroid abnormalities or chronic infections such as syphillis or
Lyme disease. One also has to rule out disorders that cause confusion
acutely, particularly liver disease, kidney disease, electrolyte abnormalities and hypoxia (lack of oxygen to the brain). Unfortunately, there are no
"biomarkers" in the blood to help us diagnose any of the major causes of
dementia. Some common ways to diagnose dementia are:

- A neurological examination may suggest certain processes.
- Specific types of gait (walking) disturbances are common in Parkinson's
  disease, vitamin B12 deficiency, normal pressure hydrocephalus or cerebrovascular disease.

- Reflex abnormalities may be seen in Creutzfeldt-Jakob disease, ALS, MS or cerebrovascular disease.

- Extrapyramidal signs (increase in tone, slowness of movement, flexed posture and decreased arm swing, diminished facial expression) occur with Parkinson's disease, Dementia with Lewy bodies and progressive supranuclear palsy.

- Problems with eye movements are present in progressive supranuclear palsy.

- Myoclonic jerks (sudden twitches of extremities or the body) can be seen in Alzheimer's disease, Creutzfeldt-Jakob disease and, rarely, in several other dementing processes.

The neurologic exam includes cognitive testing which is of paramount importance in someone having problems with thinking. If the person is severely impaired, a few questions evaluating orientation and memory may be sufficient to make a diagnosis. Also, clock drawing, delayed word recall and word list generation can often reveal if there are problems. But for evaluating a mild or moderate degree of dementia, the Folstein mini-mental state examination is probably used most frequently (see Table 1.4).[18] It consists of 11 questions that assess 5 areas of cognitive function, assigning a score to each answer. Though not a detailed evaluation, it is quick and reproducible, usually requiring 5–10 minutes, lending itself to an office practice. This can generally tell the degree of cognitive impairment present and also establishes a baseline to judge stability, deterioration or improvement in the future. The maximum score that can be obtained is 30 and a score below 23 indicates cognitive problems, adjusted for age and level of education. An intelligent, educated person who scores below 27 or 28 should make a physician suspicious.

You can see that the MMSE is very simple and one would expect high scores from intact people, unless their brains are clouded by drugs, medications, infections or some other acute problem. Removing these conditions, a low score may be indicative of dementia. Individuals with a very low IQ, mental retardation or low educational status may also do poorly in this test. Other common screening tests include the mini-cog, memory impairment screen and six item screener. The ADAS-cog (Alzheimer's disease assessment scale-cognitive subscale), which measures the core symptoms of Alzheimer's—memory, orientation, language and praxis—is good for following patients to see the progression of the disease and effects of treatment in research trials and drug studies.

Table 1.4
The Mini Mental State Examination (MMSE)

Patient
Examiner
Date

Maximum	Score	
		Orientation
5	( )	What is the (year) (season) (date) (day) (month)
5	( )	Where are we (state) (country) (town) (hospital) (floor)?
		Registration
3	( )	Name 3 objects: 1 second to say each. Then ask the patient all three after you have said them. Give one point for each correct answer. Then repeat them until patient learns all three. Count trials and record. Trials _____
		Attention and Calculation
5	( )	Subtract 7 serially from 100. 1 point for each correct answer. Stop after 5 answers. Alternatively spell "world" backward
		Recall
3	( )	Ask for the 3 objects repeated above. Give one point for each correct answer
		Language
2	( )	Name a pencil and watch
1	( )	Repeat the following: "No ifs, ands, or buts"
3	( )	Follow a three stage command: "Take a paper in your hand, fold it in half, and put it on the floor"
1	( )	Read and obey the following: CLOSE YOUR EYES
1	( )	Write a sentence
1	( )	Copy the design shown (two intersecting pentagons)
	_____	Total Score

ASSESS level of consciousness along a continuum____

Numerous other screening tests for dementia have been devised and are in use in office practices and investigational studies, some briefer and fairly reliable, and others more detailed and using different parameters for evaluation. As a general rule, none of the screening tests work well when a patient is only mildly impaired, is very intelligent or highly educated. Even though some of these individuals may have deteriorated in terms of their cognitive abilities, they may score in the normal range. A full neuropsychiatric battery of tests administered by a clinical psychologist may be required to make a more accurate diagnosis in these cases.

Imaging of the brain should be obtained in every person suspected of having dementia. Although a CT scan (computerized tomography) can he helpful, MRI scanning (magnetic resonance imaging) is of greater value. MRI scanning uses magnetic waves rather than radiation, and it may give supporting evidence for a diagnosis of Alzheimer's disease, fronto-temporal dementia, or vascular dementia, may rule out or rule in normal pressure hydrocephalus, and can eliminate the possibility of mass lesions such as a brain tumor, abscess, subdural hematoma (clots on top of the brain), and multiple sclerosis. Having a radiologist, neuro-radiologist or neurologist well versed in interpreting these studies is as important as the scan itself.

Functional MRI (fMRI) is a new technique that may be increasingly utilized in the years ahead to assess cognitive function and brain disorders. Patients are given tasks to perform involving memory, reasoning, visual recognition, etc. Then special MRI scanning techniques are employed to measure blood flow and oxygen consumption by the brain. Deficiencies may be found in specific areas of the brain in conjunction with certain tasks, the patterns indicative of particular disorders such as Alzheimer's or other dementias, assisting in the diagnosis.[19] These tests can also be used experimentally to evaluate patients and follow progression.

PET (positron emission tomography) scanning is another tool that is useful now and may be even more so in the future in assessing dementia.[20] With PET scanning, patients are given an injection of a radioactive marker, usually a form of glucose (sugar) that tends to concentrate in cells that are metabolically active. The brain is then scanned by a machine that produces pictures similar to a CT or MRI scan, but that show the relative concentration of the radioactive material in different areas. Decreased activity in the temporoparietal regions of the brain is felt to be a fairly sensitive and specific indicator of Alzheimer's disease, and in the fronto-temporal regions to be consistent with fronto-temporal dementia.

A new marker that binds to amyloid (a substance associated with Alzheimer's) is now being used experimentally for PET scans and may soon be of great clinical assistance in diagnosing dementia. Performing this type of procedure can reveal the distribution of amyloid in the brain at different stages of Alzheimer's disease while the patient is still alive. Another new compound used in PET scanning localizes in activated microglial cells (scavenger cells) in the brain that react to inflammation and clean up damaged areas. Besides aiding in diagnosis, these new techniques may allow us to assess different treatments for Alzheimer's and determine whether they are effective.

A spinal tap need not be done routinely as part of the evaluation for dementia. Though tau protein is elevated and beta-amyloid 42 decreased in the spinal fluid in Alzheimer's disease, these biomarkers do not contribute to a diagnosis since there is significant overlap in results. They are being refined however and new biomarkers being sought, so they may be more helpful in the future. Spinal taps are currently being employed mainly to exclude multiple sclerosis, inflammatory or infectious processes.

The utility of an EEG as part of the usual dementia work-up is questionable. If the presentation is atypical, or there is a suggestion of seizure activity or myoclonic jerks, an EEG may be of value.

APOE gene testing is a matter of controversy. Although we know that having the APOE 4 allele increases the risk of developing Alzheimer's, particularly if the person is a homozygous carrier, it does not mean this individual will definitely be stricken. If the test is positive, it may result in years of unnecessary anxiety or depression, since there is no intervention that can absolutely prevent Alzheimer's. On the other hand, there are many measures a person can take to reduce the risk, whether or not he or she carries the APOE 4 allele. At present, I do not recommend having this test to my patients.

Chapter 2

CONFOUNDERS OF DEMENTIA: NORMAL AGING, MILD COGNITIVE IMPAIRMENT AND PSEUDO-DEMENTIA

> Growing old is so strange because inside one feels just the same.
>
> May Sarton[1]

When physicians are asked to assess patients concerned about the possibility of dementia, they occasionally find the diagnosis uncertain. Three conditions cause much of the confusion: normal aging, mild cognitive impairment and pseudo-dementia. Even astute clinicians with years of experience can be fooled at times on either side of the equation—saying a person has early dementia when he or she does not, or saying someone does not have dementia when he or she does. Of course, with further testing or the passage of time, the fog of ambiguity dissipates and the diagnosis usually becomes clear. What is it about these three states that perplexes physicians? What are the characteristics of these three states?

NORMAL AGING

The brain can be considered man's most vital organ, for it defines who we are and allows us to interact with the world around us. The rest of the body is dedicated to serving the brain, with 20–25 percent of blood flow directed to this tiny organ which utilizes a similar amount of energy.

Processing billions of bits of information each minute, it directs our emotional responses and physical movements, in addition to being responsible for maintaining our vital functions. As with the rest of the body, normal aging produces a wide spectrum of structural changes in the brains of different individuals, and with cognitive function and behavior. Sometimes, you see men and women of 80 who look and act as if they are 50. On the other hand, you may see people who are 50, but look and act as if they are 150. It is the same way with the brain. There are a multitude of factors, genetic and environmental, that determine how our brains age, and how they are able to function. When we look at brains at autopsy, or at MRI scans, there may be considerable differences in what we are willing to call normal.

Physical and Physiologic Changes in the Brain and Nervous System

In simplified terms, the brain consists of gray matter in a mantle around the surface and in deeper islands, with white matter everywhere else. The latter is like a plant with multiple branches connecting to different areas of the gray matter, with roots running down into the spinal cord. The vast majority of neurons (nerve cells) are situated in the gray matter. These are the cells in the brain that "think," control movements and motor activity, interpret all sensory data, understand language and are able to communicate internally and with the outside world. The white matter consists of bundles of nerve fibers sheathed in a fatty material called myelin that acts as insulation. Neurons send electrical signals through their nerve fibers to other neurons, with the final gap (the synapse), from the end of the nerve fiber to the "receiving neuron," bridged by tiny packets of chemicals called neurotransmitters. When these packets are released at the end of the fiber from the "sending neuron," they transmit a message to the "receiving neuron" by acting on its cell membrane and causing changes in electrical voltage.

The brain is estimated to contain over 100 billion cells, and 20 billion neurons within the cerebral cortex.[2] Each of these neurons has an average of 7,000 synaptic connections, with each cubic centimeter of cortex containing about a trillion synapses. The average human brain at maturity weighs between 1,300 and 1,500 grams. It is smaller in women than men and encompasses about 2 percent of total body mass. (There is no correlation between brain weight and intelligence). As people age, the weight and volume of their brains decreases, with a loss of between 5 and 10 percent in their later years. This atrophy of the brain is obvious in specimens from the elderly examined at autopsy, and can be seen on CT and MRI scans. What is notable is the contraction of the gyri (the snake-like bands of tissue that make up the surface of the cortex), the widening of the sulci (the grooves between the gyri) and the dilatation of the ventricles (the cavities deep within the brain). In one study measuring brain atrophy in subjects 50 to 75 years of age, 0.4 percent of brain volume was lost each year.[3] The older a person gets, the greater the degree of atrophy expected,[4] though this can be quite variable. Individuals with diabetes have a significantly higher rate of brain atrophy. This is also true for those with a high body mass index seen in people with the so-called metabolic syndrome who are at a high risk for heart attacks and strokes as well. Heavy drinkers (two or more per day) also have increased rates of brain atrophy.

Examining the brains of older people microscopically, one finds the number of neurons in the gray matter of the cerebral cortex reduced, but not as severely as was once thought to occur. In fact, some neuroscientists believe most neurons remain healthy as we age unless affected by specific diseases. The neurons in the deep structures of the brain decrease in greater proportions and there appears to be shrinkage and loss of white matter. It was once assumed that we were born with our full compliment of neurons, and if they died or were injured, they would not regenerate or be replaced. In recent years, this belief has been modified. Given the appropriate stimulus, damaged neurons in the brain and spinal cord may be induced to regenerate. Cell division producing new neurons may also occur under some circumstances. This raises the possibility for recovery after strokes, spinal cord injuries and degenerative diseases such as Alzheimer's if we can figure out how to initiate and direct the process of repair and regeneration.

Brain cells age like miniature factories that are wearing down, with diminished output of various substances, including many proteins. Among these are enzymes and critical neurotransmitters, particularly acetylcholine and dopamine. These two chemicals, whose production dwindles, are vital to systems within the brain that control memory and motor activity (gait, movement, balance, coordination and so forth). Some of the changes seen in the elderly, such as impaired balance, flexed posture and minor problems with memory, are at least partially the result of these chemical deficiencies, though loss of neurons plays a role as well. Most likely a combination of both is responsible. There also are suggestions that genetic damage in human brains starts occurring in some people around age 40, with the genes involved in learning and memory most affected. But there are mechanisms used by brain cells that may protect the genetic material and repair damage when it occurs.

The changes at autopsy and MRI scans noted in individuals with dementia can also be seen in a normal older population. For the most part, the difference is a matter of degree, with these alterations being minor in normal older people and more pronounced in those with cognitive compromise. Thus, atrophy of the brain occurs in both groups and the pattern may be similar. Also, the amyloid plaques (senile plaques) and neurofibrillary tangles, the hallmark of Alzheimer's disease, can be found in normal older brains, even in people with none of the symptoms of Alzheimer's. In addition, tiny vascular changes in the white matter that are ubiquitous in dementia are present as well in normal people.

It has been said that as we age we lose intelligence but gain wisdom. What is meant by this is that even though some of our neurons die off, the connections between the ones remaining (synapses) increase, and so more pathways between cells are developed. The dendrites (branches) of surviving neurons, where the synapses are located, expand in the normal aging brain.[5] New synapses continue to arise as a result of new experiences that have been filtered through our sensory systems and modulate the way we react to events. Wisdom can be thought of as accumulated experience that allows older individuals to make sound judgements, though they may not arrive at decisions as rapidly as younger men and women. In days past, the elderly were revered as "sages" because of their perceptiveness, balanced world views and experience: the wisdom that only comes with age.

The increased time required to perform various cognitive tasks is a major consequence of aging. Processing new information just takes longer, learning takes longer and reaction to various stimuli takes longer. Though central processing in the brain is slower, learning can certainly occur and most tasks can be accomplished. As the scientist Leonard Hayflick noted—"Loss of mental capacity with age is not inevitable. The old idea that senility is a normal accompaniment of age is simply wrong."[6]

Memory is another function that declines with age, starting to become evident in our fifties. Episodic, short-term memory is most affected, while long-term and working memory may remain remarkably intact in many older people. Often, individuals will block a word, a name or a particular event, and it comes back to them seconds or hours later. This may become more pronounced with each succeeding decade, but is a normal occurrence, and though frustrating, is not disabling. Some use the term "age related memory loss" or "age related forgetfulness" or "age associated cognitive decline" to describe what is happening. They do not indicate that dementia is right around the corner. In community studies, 25–50 percent of individuals over the age of 65 reported subjective memory loss.[7] But these people do not appear to be at increased risk of developing dementia unless testing corroborates that problems with memory truly exist.

Our sensory systems also fail as we grow older, making life more difficult because of interference with our ability to gather information. Vision may not be as acute due to cataracts, glaucoma or macular degeneration. Hearing may decline due to problems with the auditory apparatus or deterioration of the auditory nerves. Similarly, our senses of smell, taste and touch are affected. In addition to these peripheral mechanisms faltering with age, central integration and analysis of the sensory data may be deficient. Whatever the reasons, we are not getting the same amount of sensory input that was once available to us, further weakening our capacity to react rapidly to situations.

The systems that control motor function also deteriorate with aging, affecting balance and coordination, muscle strength, gait and fluidity of movement. This interferes with performance of motor tasks and reduces stamina. Although cognition is not directly impacted, it may lead to increased fatigue, or even depression, with difficulty in concentration and execution of complex mental endeavors.

Normal aging, with loss of brain cells, may release personality traits present previously, but held in check. This may also be seen in mild cognitive impairment, and is generally more subtle than the behavioral disturbances found in frank dementia. As examples of exaggerated personality traits, a person who has always been tense and suspicious of other people may become extremely guarded and watchful when older, and paranoid if demented. Or someone who has been jocular and outgoing may become more boisterous and unrestrained in later years.

With all the obstacles seemingly in place before us as we age, degrading our ability to think and perceive the world around us, one would imagine that all older people would be demented, or at the very least have severe cognitive difficulties. We know this to be far from the truth, with the majority of seniors remaining independent and functioning at a high level. In addition to managing their own lives, many older individuals continue to accomplish great things creatively, in business, in politics, in science and numerous other fields, showing that their minds are working more than adequately. Some are able to perform as well, or even better than younger individuals in their own disciplines. As examples, in the arts we know that Picasso and Chagall were painting into their nineties, Saul Bellow was writing novels and Arthur Miller plays in their late eighties, with Toscanini conducting and Horowitz giving piano concerts in their ninth decades.

Studies have shown that older animals and people can learn and preserve intelligence given the right environments.[8] Behavioral enrichment and mental stimulation together with a diet fortified with antioxidants enhanced the ability of dogs to learn and appeared to slow age-dependant cognitive decline. In humans, an intellectually challenging life (and various other activities we will detail later) allows us to combat the effects of aging on our brains. Although we may not be able to paint like Picasso, or write like Saul Bellow when we are in our eighties, most of us can learn new material, think logically and manage our own lives.

How Normal Aging can be Mistaken for Dementia

Older people may move and respond more slowly, and at times this delay may be equated with deficiencies in thinking and judgement. This can be compounded when a person has impaired vision or hearing. A question may be answered inappropriately, or the answer may not make sense, simply because it was not heard correctly and the person was replying to a different query. Similarly, behavior may seem strange or improper, because the individual was acting in a different context, resulting from a different interpretation of the situation due to visual or hearing compromise. This is not an unusual occurrence and has to be considered before diagnosing dementia, particularly if the person lives alone and appears to have no problems in handling the tasks of daily living.

Case History (Normal Aging)

Martha was a 73-year-old woman, impeccably dressed, who came to my office concerned about problems with memory. This had been present for about two years, though she was unsure of the actual onset and whether it had progressed. A college graduate, she had been employed in a managerial job for a while, but had retired 20 years earlier. She did some volunteer work and was active in a few art-related groups. She lived with her husband, who was 10 years older than she and disabled by severe heart disease, in a large house. With no significant medical or family history, she exercised daily and took care of every aspect of her own and her husband's lives. She had no problems driving or balancing her checkbook, but occasionally missed appointments and had difficulty remembering names. At times, she might enter a room for something, then forget what it was. Usually, this would come back to her shortly. Neurologic examination was completely normal and she scored 29 of 30 on the MMSE, recalling only two of three objects she was asked to remember. Her MRI was essentially normal for her age with some minor small vessel changes in the white matter. Formal neuropsychological testing revealed no deficits.

I thought the patient might be slightly depressed because of the situation with her husband and suggested she take a mild antidepressant in addition to a baby aspirin to prevent strokes and improve blood flow to the brain. She agreed to the aspirin, but did not want to take the antidepressant. Over the next several years, she was seen at six monthly intervals, still complaining of problems with memory, though on brief testing in the office she did fine. Then she stopped coming, returning 4 years later because of neck pain. Her husband had died in the interim, she had sold the house and was now living alone and functioning well. She still insisted her memory was impaired, though nothing was found on testing. Eight years after the initial consultation, she remained intact and able to handle the tasks of daily living.

MILD COGNITIVE IMPAIRMENT (MCI)

Though mild cognitive impairment has been recognized for the past decade or so, there is considerable debate over whether it should be considered an actual entity, with some neurologists believing it to be early stage of dementia and others feeling there is no need for this label.[9] The question is whether this is a pathological state, or simply a pattern of normal aging. Because the criteria at different centers diagnosing this condition vary, patients are far from uniform and it is felt that standardization of methodology is necessary.[10] If the diagnostic guidelines recommended by the American Academy of Neurology are used, individuals with MCI are not normal, but are also not demented. While many individuals with MCI do progress to dementia, others remain stable and some may even improve. Certainly those with MCI are at increased risk for dementia and should be carefully monitored.

There have been suggestions that there are two main groups of patients with MCI who differ in presentation, pathologic changes and progression.[11] The amnestic group (those with mostly memory problems) have less white matter changes on their MRIs (usually due to diminished blood flow in the small blood vessels), elevated levels of tau protein in their spinal fluid (a marker of Alzheimer's), and are more likely to convert to Alzheimer's over time. The second group of patients with more generalized impairment of cognitive function have more changes in the white matter of their brains, but do not progress to dementia and remain cognitively stable over a two-year period. Their decline in intellectual ability is felt to be more likely on a vascular basis, than as a precursor of Alzheimer's. Unfortunately, a greater proportion of MCI patients appear to have the amnestic form of the disorder.

Labeling someone as having mild cognitive impairment is determined by history, neurologic examination and neuropsychological evaluation, with no specific laboratory tests that aid in making a diagnosis. Changes on MRIs are nonspecific with varying degrees of atrophy and white matter changes, and nothing in the blood or spinal fluid that is helpful. Medial temporal lobe atrophy on MRI may be predictive of which patients will develop Alzheimer's.[12] Special imaging such as fMRI and PET may also have some predictive value.

The term mild cognitive impairment connotes a transitional stage between normal aging and dementia, with MMSE scores generally in the range of 24–28 (top score is 30). However, individuals with high levels of educational or intellectual achievement may score from 28–30 and still be cognitively impaired. Formal neuropsychometric testing that takes previous mental capacity into consideration may be better able to delineate when cognitive decline has occurred. The current criteria for a diagnosis of mild cognitive impairment are given below (see Table 2.1). At times, however, even with use of these guidelines it may be difficult to differentiate between normal aging and MCI, or between MCI and early dementia.

Table 2.1
Criteria for Mild Cognitive Impairment

Memory complaint, preferably corroborated by an informant
Objective memory impairment for age and education
Largely intact general cognitive function
Essentially preserved activities of daily living
Not demented[a]

---

[a]R.C. Peterson et al., "Mild cognitive impairment. Clinical characterization and outcome," *Arch Neurol*, 1999, 56: 303–308.

It was initially believed that memory loss greater than expected in normal aging was characteristic of MCI, with other cognitive parameters remaining fairly intact. Affected individuals did not meet the established guidelines for dementia, as they were able to live by themselves and manage their own affairs. However, some studies have suggested a global decline in cognitive function in people with MCI (even the amnestic type) and not just memory alone. And we know that individuals having MCI do progress to dementia at an elevated rate compared to healthy age-matched controls, particularly those people with the amnestic form. Some neurologists have suggested that over 5 to 6 years, about 85 percent of patients with MCI will develop Alzheimer's disease.[13] Conversion rates of 12–20 percent annually have been found, compared to 1–2 percent in a normal population of similar age. But other neuroscientists feel that a much lower percentage of patients with MCI eventually develop Alzheimer's. The criteria used to make a diagnosis and the setting where the patients are seen may be responsible for some of the differences, with university-based practices having higher rates of conversion. Autopsy studies of people diagnosed with MCI (particularly the amnestic type) who have died from other causes do have the pathologic features of Alzheimer's disease.

If ways could be found to arrest the progression of MCI, or even reverse the process, many individuals and families would be rescued from sinking into the quicksand of dementia, along with the heartache and despair that accompanies the descent. The involved individuals could live independently longer with a more satisfactory quality of life. In addition, the health care system would save billions of dollars that could be put to other use. It would help if we could predict which MCI patients were most likely to develop Alzheimer's, and different possible markers for this are being investigated. Regarding therapy, there have been suggestions that programs that intensively stimulate cognitive function and certain motor activities on a long-term basis may stabilize the deterioration in MCI and mild Alzheimer's while also improving patients' mood, at least temporarily.[14] Additional work needs to be done in this area.

A number of studies are also in progress to see whether various medications can halt the conversion of MCI to dementia. One recent report showed that Donepezil, a treatment for Alzheimer's disease, delayed the progression of the amnestic form of MCI to Alzheimer's for about a year, but at the end of three years, there was no significant difference.[15] Giving 2,000 IU of vitamin E daily to patients with MCI produced no benefits at all. The rate of progression from MCI to dementia in this study was

16 percent per year over a 3-year period. Another study suggested that a subgroup of MCI patients with an elevated chemical in the blood called homocysteine (a risk factor for heart attacks, strokes and dementia) might be stabilized by taking a combination of vitamin B12, vitamin B6 and folate, but this needs to be investigated further.[16] There are no hard recommendations at this time in terms of treating MCI with any specific medications, but the search continues for a substance or substances that will halt or reverse ongoing decline.

Case History (MCI)

Liz was an 81-year-old woman with severe heart disease who came for evaluation because she and her husband were concerned about her inability to remember things. Her husband was present during the interview and examination, often answering questions before she had a chance to speak. Finishing two years of college, she had stayed at home after marriage to raise three children. Subsequently, she been active in her church, had spent time playing golf, and visiting her children and grandchildren. The problems with memory were first noted about a year earlier, shortly after she had an angioplasty (a cardiac procedure) to open a partially blocked coronary artery. Her husband believed it had gotten slightly worse since then, though she was uncertain. She was able to drive locally without getting lost, did all the cooking, and they shared household chores. He had always done the checkbook and paid the bills. Since her difficulty had begun, she occasionally misplaced things in the house, forgot appointments and people's names, and at times neglected to take various medications. She had a borderline blood pressure and cholesterol in addition to her heart condition. On examination, she was fully oriented, knew the president and vice president and had a fairly good fund of knowledge. She was able to calculate well and could spell WORLD backward. But given three objects to remember, she could recall none of them after five minutes. And when given them again, she remembered one five minutes later. Her neurologic exam was otherwise intact aside from minor problems with balance.

Formal neuropsychological testing revealed considerable problems with memory and some loss of function in other areas. She was not demented however, being able to fully care for herself and carry on the tasks of daily living. The clinical psychologist confirmed a diagnosis of mild cognitive impairment. MRI showed atrophy commensurate with age and extensive white matter vascular changes.

The patient was already on aspirin and this was continued. Her primary care physician was also advised to treat her cholesterol and blood pressure more aggressively to see if this might arrest her cognitive decline. Unfortunately, during the next two years there was further deterioration and it was evident she had crossed the line into dementia. No longer able to drive by herself without getting lost, she also required help in planning and preparing meals. She was started on the medication Donepezil, which is used to treat Alzheimer's, and over a nine-month period has remained stable.

PSEUDO-DEMENTIA

Pseudo-dementia (false or imitation dementia) was a term originally used by neurologists as a description for psychiatric illnesses that masqueraded as dementia. The most common of these was depression and schizophrenia. Though these illnesses may present diagnostic dilemmas for physicians at times, a number of other conditions can be mistaken for dementia as well.

Psychiatric Illnesses

Depression is widespread in our older population and at times can be confused with dementia. Not every depressed person will be thought to be demented, since most often the diagnosis is straightforward. But in a small percentage of cases it is unclear what is wrong. This is more likely to happen in patients with major depressions, who are apathetic, respond slowly, are inattentive, have difficulty learning and can have problems with memory and executive function. It must also be remembered that depression and dementia often coexist, and people who are cognitively impaired may be depressed as well. In addition, it was previously mentioned that depression may predispose individuals to dementia. Thus, it may take a very astute clinician to decide whether depression or dementia is the primary problem. A good history from the family may be very helpful in distinguishing between the two conditions, and the observations that relatives make can be critical. At times, neuropsychological testing can be of assistance as well. When a definite diagnosis cannot be established, treatment for depression may be indicated since the process may potentially be ameliorated or reversed. But interestingly, successful therapy for depression does not exclude the possibility of an underlying early dementia.

Schizophrenia can sometimes be mistaken for dementia as well. Hallucinations, language problems and strange behavior can occur in both conditions along with impaired executive function and learning difficulty. The key here is the age of the affected person. Schizophrenia is seen most often early in life: in the teenage years, twenties and perhaps thirties. It rarely starts later on. On the other hand, dementia predominantly attacks older people and would be quite unusual in the decades when schizophrenia is prevalent.

Case History (Pseudo-Dementia)

Alice, a 62-year-old woman with difficulty functioning for about five months, was brought to me by her husband, having been referred by their internist who thought she was demented. The physician had obtained routine blood work which was normal. An MRI was pending. During this period, she had become withdrawn and apathetic, had stopped taking care of the house and preparing meals. She rarely initiated conversation though she would respond when spoken to. Her husband said she did not seem to remember things he told her. Much of her day was spent in a bathrobe watching television, yet she didn't seem to recall what she had seen. There was a history of a severe depressive episode requiring hospitalization 25 years earlier after a miscarriage, but there had been no problems after that. For many years, she smoked two packs of cigarettes daily and ingested large amounts of coffee. Never having graduated from high school, she had worked in various retail jobs and as a waitress, though not in the past 7 years. This was her third marriage. She had three children from her first one, none of whom lived nearby.

On neurologic examination, she moved and reacted deliberately. She knew the month but not the year nor which town she was in. On three attempts, she could recall none of three objects she was told to remember, but didn't appear to be paying much attention. She had no language problems or difficulty following instructions, except for the length of time it took her to react. Aside from the simplest sums, calculations could not be performed. Testing of motor skills, balance and coordination, reflexes, sensation and cranial nerves were all normal, as was her blood pressure.

It was not clear to me on my first encounter whether she was demented, or had a major depression, or perhaps both. Her MRI showed small vessel changes, perhaps slightly more than what would be expected for her age, but no significant atrophy. An EEG was essentially normal. Neuropsychological testing was not ordered, as it was felt she would be unable to cooperate. She was started on an antidepressant and a psychiatric consultation was obtained. The psychiatrist was also uncertain about the diagnosis, but thought it would be worthwhile continuing the treatment for depression, and he increased her dosage substantially. Initially, it did not seem to make any difference, but as he added other medications over a four-to-five-week period, she began to improve. Eventually, she returned almost to her baseline, but had to be maintained on medications.

Fixed Cognitive Deficits

Mental retardation and low intelligence levels can only be mistaken for dementia if a history is unavailable. Since the cognitive difficulties have existed from an early age and are static, the diagnosis should be clear cut. Similarly, traumatic brain injuries (TBI) that have occurred previously and produced fixed deficits should present no quandaries in terms of diagnosis.

Cerebral hypoxia or anoxia (lack of oxygen to the brain) can also be responsible for cognitive impairment which is generally static. Any process that results in decreased oxygen supply to the brain (cardiac arrest, bleeding ulcers, chronic obstructive pulmonary disease, anesthesia problems, carbon monoxide poisoning) can cause brain damage and death of neurons. But once this has occurred, the intellectual problems usually do not progress, unless compromise in the oxygen supply is repeated.

Acute Cognitive Impairment

An acute "organic brain syndrome" (OBS), confusional state or delirium is usually not mistaken for dementia because of its rapid onset and lack of chronicity. Acute problems that produce an "organic brain syndrome" are most often the result of intoxication, or metabolic abnormalities. Physical examination and testing of the blood or urine frequently provides a diagnosis. Older people, whose complement of neurons is already diminished, are much more susceptible to cognitive difficulties when their remaining cells are stressed by any process that upsets the normal chemical balance of the blood and the cells. Electrolyte disturbances involving high or low levels of sodium, potassium, calcium, chloride or bicarbonate can all cause acute "organic brain syndromes" which is manifest as a delirium or confusional state. Once the electrolyte imbalance is corrected, normal brain function generally returns. Liver disease with high ammonia levels and kidney disease with elevated urea and creatinine levels (a substance excreted in the urine) also cause acute "organic brain syndromes." All of these conditions together can also be categorized under the heading of metabolic encephalopathies—impaired brain function due to metabolic abnormalities.

The older brain is also particularly vulnerable to drugs and alcohol, resulting in greater sedation, confusion and problems with balance when these substances enter the neuronal environment in more than minimal amounts. While these difficulties usually disappear when the substances are broken down and metabolized, chronic use of large amounts of alcohol and various drugs can cause brain cells to die and result in permanent dysfunction. Prescribed medications can also affect the brain adversely in lower doses than younger people are able to tolerate, producing confusional states. In the elderly, the liver and kidneys do not work as effectively to metabolize foreign substances as they once did. Thus, medications, drugs and alcohol may accumulate in higher amounts than expected and disrupt brain cells.

There has also been a recent report that steroids can produce dementia.[17] Previously, steroids were known to cause psychosis, but dementia can also develop. Fortunately, this is rapidly reversible when steroids are discontinued.

Infections such as pneumonia or urinary tract infections can cause confusion in older people even though the brain is not directly impacted. The fever from these conditions heightens metabolic demands on brain cells that they are unable to meet, causing the impairment. Shortly after the fever breaks, underlying brain function is usually restored and the confusion disappears.

Illnesses such as meningitis (an infection of the covering of the brain) and encephalitis (an infection of brain tissue) result in confusional states and disturbed thinking that generally improve when the infections are controlled. However, permanent brain damage can also occur, producing static deficits. In some types of encephalitis (herpes), short-term memory may be preferentially destroyed because of the severity of temporal lobe and hippocampal involvement. The affected person may live the rest of his or her life with no return of function, usually limited to the obliteration of memory.

There is also a syndrome (condition) known as transient global amnesia (TGA) which presents as a sudden loss of short-term memory. This impairment lasts a brief period of time, usually hours, rarely days, and then clears. Individuals with TGA cannot remember anything that happens during the period they are affected, and may ask the same questions over and over again, forgetting the answers received moments before.

Even when this disturbance passes and they return to normal, they are unaware of what took place during the time they were impaired. People with TGA could be mistaken for Alzheimer's patients if the observer did not realize the memory loss had come on suddenly and was going to pass soon afterward. The cause of this condition is unknown, but it is hypothesized that there is transient compromise of the arterial circulation, or venous congestion in areas of the brain responsible for short-term memory (hippocampus and medial temporal lobe), resulting in temporary malfunction. Recently, a special type of MRI study (diffusion weighted imaging or DWI) has been able to demonstrate abnormalities in the hippocampus 24 to 48 hours after the onset of symptoms.[18]

It was mentioned previously that traumatic brain injuries can cause brain damage that remains fixed. A cerebral concussion can produce cognitive problems acutely, particularly loss of memory, but also impaired concentration and global difficulties with mental tasks. These problems may linger as part of a post-concussion syndrome with headaches and dizziness that passes over time. Sometime, it may take months or even longer for recovery. A portion of these patients can be left with long-term minor deficits, but not enough to be considered demented.

Chapter 3

ALZHEIMER'S DISEASE

The simplest reality appears to change.

Te Tao Ching[1]

An idle mind is the devil's workshop
And the devil is Alzheimer's.

George Carlin riff

Aside from cancer, the illness people most fear as they age is Alzheimer's disease, a progressive neurodegenerative condition that is ultimately fatal, its incidence increasing with each year of life. It attacks both rich and poor, and all races, and does not respect fame nor power. Ronald Reagan succumbed to its onslaught as did Rita Hayworth. Many people think of Alzheimer's as being equivalent to dementia, and, indeed, it is the most common cause. Because it is ubiquitous in the elderly population, virtually all older persons know someone stricken by this disorder and are familiar with its effects on memory, cognitive function and quality of life. They live in mortal dread that this phantom will attack them as well, and they will lose their minds and control of their lives.

Currently, the number of people in America estimated to have Alzheimer's disease is about 4 to 4.5 million,[2] and it is estimated that this number could triple or even quadruple by the year 2050 if no cure or preventative is discovered. Twenty to thirty million people worldwide are currently believed to be affected.[3] The disease is present in 1 percent of people at 60 years of age and 30 to 40 percent of those 85 years old. About 50 to 75 percent of all cases of dementia are due to Alzheimer's disease, alone or in combination with other processes, such as vascular disease, Lewy body disease, or both. Alzheimer's takes a tremendous financial toll on individuals and society, and the emotional consequences on victims' families are immeasurable. Thirty-four percent of the Medicare budget goes for the care of Alzheimer's patients, though they represent only 13 percent of the population over 65. The Alzheimer's Association in 2005 estimated that caring for an individual with Alzheimer's costs an average of $174,000 for the duration of the disease. A significant percentage of patients with Alzheimer's are not diagnosed or misdiagnosed, 40 percent in one study,[4] and 50 percent of those diagnosed are not treated. Many investigators feel the true numbers are even higher.

Though Alzheimer's disease is one of the most frequent conditions seen by physicians today, particularly neurologists and geriatricians, it was barely recognized and poorly understood 30 to 50 years ago. In 1973, *Merritt's Textbook of Neurology*, a standard and perhaps preeminent textbook of the time, described Alzheimer's disease as a rare condition.[5] Two other important textbooks of neurology—Sir Francis Walshe's *Diseases of the Nervous System*, published in 1958, and Lord Brain's *Diseases of the Nervous System*, published in 1962—do not even mention Alzheimer's in their pages as a common disorder that neurologists must be knowledgeable about.[6] The symptoms of Alzheimer's in the elderly were simply dismissed as senility: an expected occurrence in older people.

Alzheimer's disease was first described in 1906 by Dr. Alois Alzheimer, a German neurologist, in a 51-year-old woman. Initially, this was categorized as "pre-senile" dementia, with the cognitive decline occurring earlier in life than the naturally expected dementia of the elderly. Pick's disease (fronto-temporal dementia) was lumped together with Alzheimer's in many treatises on the subject, the belief being this was justified because their clinical pictures were so similar.[7] Subsequently these two conditions were found to be different, and it was also found that the disease process in Alzheimer's was the same in younger people as in the elderly. This eliminated the so-called presenile dementia. Eventually, it was decided that the condition is not normal even later in life.

The clinical picture of Alzheimer's includes progressive impairment of memory, problems with language, difficulties with spatial orientation, deterioration in executive function, judgment and decision-making, and problems with learning new information or tasks. Behavioral disturbances are also common. These cognitive abnormalities are due to the deposition of a proteinaceous material in the brain called amyloid, which aggregates into so-called senile plaques, and a substance known as tau protein that forms neurofibrillary tangles within the neurons. However, people do not meet the criteria for Alzheimer's, or any dementia, unless their impairment is great enough to prevent independent living and managing of their own lives.

GENETICS OF ALZHEIMER'S DISEASE

For most of the cases of Alzheimer's that occur later in life, the genetic pattern is extremely complex and yet to be fully elucidated. True familial Alzheimer's disease encompasses less than 10 percent of total patients with this disorder,[8] and can be subdivided further into those patients who develop the disease before and after age 65: early onset and late onset. The familial type of Alzheimer's manifesting early in life has been shown to be associated with specific mutations on chromosomes 21, 14 and 1. Late onset familial Alzheimer's is associated with APOE 4 coding on chromosome 19. All the forms of familial Alzheimer's have an autosomal dominant pattern of inheritance, which means they can be passed on by one parent alone. Two genes that are closely related (the presenilins PSEN1 and PSEN2) have been connected to the autosomal dominant form of Alzheimer's that occurs prior to age 65: what was once called presenile dementia. This is mainly linked to PSEN1 which seems to produce a more virulent form of the disease. Currently, 142 mutations have been discovered in PSEN1 and 10 in PSEN2. The initial genetic defect responsible for Alzheimer's was found on the amyloid precursor protein gene (APP) on chromosome 21. Subsequently, more than 23 different mutations and gene linkages involving amyloid precursor protein have been detected. However, these make up only a small percentage of the total cases of familial Alzheimer's.

The genetic pattern APOE 4, either one or two copies of the gene, is a significant risk factor for the development of Alzheimer's disease in the sporadic and late onset forms. Homozygosity (two copies of the gene) in Alzheimer's patients is associated with an earlier age of onset, greater amounts of amyloid deposits and lower levels of the neurotransmitter acetylcholine. Though many other genes appear to increase susceptibility to Alzheimer's, in both the early onset and late onset forms, the exact manner in which they exert influence is not always clear. But APOE 4 is the most important and widespread genetic factor related to this disorder. About 15–25 percent of the general population carry the APOE 4 gene, though only a portion of them will develop Alzheimer's. Carrying the gene, even two copies, does not guarantee a person will be stricken. It just increases his or her chances, even more so for those who are homozygous. On the other hand, having the APOE 2 or APOE 3 genes offers some protection and reduces the risk.

Since the evolution of Alzheimer's in different people having the same complement of genes is so variable, it is evident that environmental factors must be important in determining if and when and how an individual gets the disease. This means there are elements of the process we may be able to control. As one example, it appears that APOE 4 carriers who have coexisting cerebrovascular disease are more likely to acquire Alzheimer's disease than those who don't.[9] And measures that diminish atherosclerosis and cerebrovascular disease can lower the chances of developing Alzheimer's.

PATHOLOGY AND POSSIBLE CAUSES OF ALZHEIMER'S DISEASE

Currently, the dominant theory regarding the cause of Alzheimer's disease is the amyloid cascade hypothesis. This theory proposes that amyloid precursor protein (APP) is broken down by various enzymes (gamma- and beta-secretases) to generate beta-amyloid 42 fibrils and senile plaques in the brain. These fibrils and plaques are toxic to neurons and produce an inflammatory reaction that causes cell damage and eventual destruction of synapses and neurons. Neurofibrillary tangles form as a result of destabilization of the microtubules within the neurons. Transmission of impulses between neurons at the synapses becomes increasingly impaired, particularly in the cholinergic system (the neurons that use acetylcholine as a neurotransmitter) which is important in memory. The increase in beta-amyloid 42 in the brains of Alzheimer's patients could occur because of heightened production (due to increased activity of gamma- and beta-secretases), or because of a reduction in the breakdown and clearance. APOE is involved in some way with regulating the degradation and clearance of amyloid from the brain and may also be responsible for transforming beta-amyloid into toxic fibrils.

An alternative theory that has recently gained traction posits that the damage in Alzheimer's is initiated by a soluble form of beta-amyloid 42 called ADDLs (Amyloid beta Derived Diffusable Ligands) rather than the amyloid plaques and fibrils. The latter are generated during the later stages of the disease and are not responsible for the early symptoms. ADDLs may also produce the memory loss in amnestic mild cognitive impairment which progresses to Alzheimer's in such a high percentage. The soluble ADDLs cause abnormal signaling at the synapses between the neurons and synaptic failure, creating the familiar clinical picture of Alzheimer's, but not neuronal death. A progression can be envisioned with the accumulation of small fragments of beta-amyloid 42 called monomers, oligomers and polymers that combine in larger assemblies and cause synaptic and dendritic dysfunction, with activation of inflammatory cells in the brain (microglia and astrocytes).[10] This is followed by various other changes in the cells and extracellular environment, including free radical formation, oxidative injury, neuronal impairment and eventually death. This theory holds that Alzheimer's is a disease of synaptic failure—an information storage disease. If this hypothesis is valid, it provides new targets for treatment. These include blocking the assembly of ADDLs from small fragments, blocking their effects on the receptor sites in the synapses where ADDLs cause disruption or attacking ADDLs directly with specific antibodies.

A protein called insulin-degrading enzyme (IDE) appears to play a role in amyloid clearance from the brain, and insulin itself may enhance the formation of beta-amyloid protein or inhibit its degradation.[11] In fact another hypothesis has been advanced proposing that Alzheimer's is a neuroendocrine disease, perhaps Type 3 Diabetes, involving insulin and insulin-like growth factor (IGF) which are essential for neuronal survival.[12] Insulin has been shown to be produced in the brain and there are insulin receptors there as well. Abnormalities may be present in insulin signaling and regulation, but the mechanism of how this results in the pathologic changes of Alzheimer's is yet to be elucidated. A recent study found that heightened levels of insulin in the blood "can elevate inflammatory markers and beta-amyloid 42 in the periphery and the brain, thereby potentially increasing the risk of Alzheimer's disease."[13]

Pathologically, the brains of patients with Alzheimer's at autopsy are atrophied. The most prominent changes initially involve the structures of the medial temporal lobe, particularly the body of cells called the hippocampus, and the entorhinal cortex. Eventually, there is atrophy of the entire cerebral cortex and dilatation of the ventricles of the brain (the internal cavities). Microscopically, the neuritic plaques, also known as senile plaques, which occur outside the brain cells, and the neurofibrillary tangles intracellularly (within the cells), are characteristic of Alzheimer's. The senile plaques are formed by deposits of amyloid resulting from the breakdown of amyloid precursor protein, producing beta-amyloid 40 and beta-amyloid 42. Both forms of amyloid are toxic, but the latter much more so. Though beta-amyloid 42 comprises only 5–20 percent of the total beta-amyloid, it constitutes about 50 percent of amyloid in the senile plaques. The neurofibrillary tangles consist of a type of protein called tau, which comes from the microtubules within the cell, that has been changed chemically (hyperphosphoralation). Early in the course of the disease, the plaques and tangles are most evident in the hippocampus and medial temporal lobe, but are seen throughout the brain as the disease progresses. Over time as well, the damaged neurons begin to die and less brain cells are available to respond to any treatment that may be given. Synaptic transmission between neurons is also affected by these changes, particularly with acetylcholine, though all neurotransmitters are involved. These patients have what is known as a cholinergic deficit—a major decrease in the amount of acetyl-choline available to transmit impulses between nerve cells, with a loss of the enzyme ChAT (choline acetyltransferase) that makes acetylcholine.

The various symptoms we associate with the disease are the result of these chemical and cellular changes. In the amyloid cascade theory, there is a suggestion that the early manifestations of Alzheimer's are associated mainly with an increase in amyloid (senile) plaques, particularly in the hippocampus, while the later symptoms are correlated with the more extensive appearance of neurofibrillary tangles.[14] However, a number of studies have shown that the degree of cognitive impairment in an individual does not correlate with the characteristic pathologic findings at autopsy, and that synaptic loss is a much better indicator of the severity of the dementia that had been present.[15] Indeed, neuronal injury and synaptic dysfunction may exist for decades before neuronal death occurs, emphasizing that an effective therapy may have to begin very early in the course of the disease.

DIAGNOSING ALZHEIMER'S DISEASE

When diagnosing Alzheimer's disease, it must be differentiated from mild cognitive impairment, other forms of dementia and rarely from pseudo-dementia (see Table 3.1). Separating the amnestic form of MCI from early Alzheimer's can be difficult and may be merely a semantic exercise, because the vast majority of these individuals go on to develop Alzheimer's anyway. It may be important, however, in terms of when to start treatment, particularly when more effective therapies are available in the future. Currently, the arbitrary line dividing MCI from Alzheimer's disease is the ability of the individual to function independently. Unless the condition is more advanced, MMSE testing may not be able to provide a definitive answer, particularly if the person were highly intelligent or educated, making extensive neuropsychological testing necessary. The early diagnosis of Alzheimer's may also be essential because of safety issues, such as driving and cooking, and to be certain that advanced planning is handled while the person is relatively intact.

Table 3.1
Criteria for the Diagnosis of Probable Alzheimer's Disease

Typical history of Alzheimer's disease
Insidious onset of symptoms
Gradual progression of symptoms
Cognitive loss documented by cognitive tests
No physical signs or neuroimaging or laboratory evidence of other diseases
    that could cause dementia (such as strokes, Parkinson's disease, subdural
    hematoma, or tumors.)[a]

---

[a]The criteria are consistent with the National Institute of Neurologic and Communicative Disorders and Stroke- Alzheimer's Disease and Related Disorders Association (NINCDS-ADRDA) criteria.
Source: Clauda Kawas, "Early Alzheimer's Disease," *N Eng J Med* (2003), 349: 1056–1063

In evaluating someone with possible Alzheimer's, the starting point is the history taken from the patient and his or her family to track the sequence and severity of the intellectual difficulties, while also looking for any depressive symptoms. This is followed by a neurologic examination, including cognitive screening tests. There are then specific blood studies searching for uncommon causes of dementia, and an MRI. Formal neuropsychological testing may be next in selected patients. Whether an EEG, spinal tap, PET scan and other more specialized studies are done depends on the person's clinical picture. APOE profiling is not obtained routinely.

A good history may be sufficient to make a diagnosis even prior to cognitive testing. The onset of the disease is usually insidious with the family becoming aware of a problem with memory and judgment over a period of years, or many months. At times, there may be a precipitating event that brings the patient to a physician's attention, such as the family's concern over mom or dad getting lost while driving. Being overdrawn at the bank, an inability to reconcile the checkbook or other difficulties with finances may sometimes be the final straw for a spouse or the children. In addition, missing appointments, missing medications, or neglecting personal hygiene or care of the household, may make the family realize something is amiss. Another frequent symptom is the inability to operate household appliances—from cable television and VCRs to washing machines and stoves. Forgetting to turn off the oven, or a burner on the stove can occasionally result in disaster. The deterioration in the person's cognitive abilities progresses gradually, and at times almost imperceptibly, as the downward spiral continues. Occasionally, a plateau in functioning may be seen that is maintained for awhile before the descent resumes. Patients rarely have insight into what is happening, though they may know that things are not quite right, with difficulty expressing what that is. At times, this vague unease may be manifested by depression, or feelings of anxiety. Denial by the family that a problem exists is not uncommon, until matters get out of hand. Spouses or children are reluctant to admit to themselves that a loved one is demented, with everything that encompasses from an emotional standpoint, financial responsibilities and time commitments.

Apart from cognitive testing, the neurologic and physical examinations are usually normal. As mentioned previously, carriers of the APOE 4 gene are much more prone to developing Alzheimer's, particularly those who are homozygous, but its presence does not substantiate a diagnosis. At present, there are no specific blood tests that aid in diagnosis.

On MRI, the classic finding is atrophy of the hippocampus and medial temporal lobes. Not infrequently, however, there may be widespread atrophy throughout the entire cerebral cortex. Vascular changes in the white matter of the brain, noted to some degree in most older people, are also seen in those with Alzheimer's. While this finding predisposes individuals to dementia if extensive, it does not have particular significance in terms of diagnosis.

There are no specific EEG abnormalities, but the test should be done if the patient has seizures or seizure-like activity, which can be induced by the disease process. The EEG may be normal or show mild slowing if no seizure discharges are present.

PET (photon emission tomography) scanning may be quite helpful in diagnosing problem cases of Alzheimer's,[16] but currently is not employed routinely. It is difficult for physicians to convince insurance companies of the utility of the procedure and have them pay for it. New techniques enhance PETs value even more if C-PIB, a biomarker for amyloid, is utilized. SPECT scanning may also be of assistance in some cases.

Though tau protein (from neurofibrillary tangles) is increased in the spinal fluid of patients with Alzheimer's, and beta-amyloid 42 is decreased, the findings are sufficiently ambiguous to negate the use of spinal taps as part of the customary evaluation. In addition to tau protein and beta-amyloid 42, the other so-called biomarkers of Alzheimer's in spinal fluid include phospho-tau (also from neurofibrillary tangles) and isoprotanes (an indicator of inflammation). A new test, which is still experimental, is able to detect ADDLs in spinal fluid and may become an important biomarker in the future.[17] Studies are also being done to see whether it is possible to find ADDLs in the blood and perhaps use this as a test for Alzheimer's. Other possible blood biomarkers being investigated are beta-amyloid 42/beta-amyloid 40 ratios, and the level of a neurosteroid called 3 alpha, 5 alpha-THP which may play a role in learning, memory and synaptic function.

Formal neuropsychological testing can be of great assistance in diagnosing Alzheimer's or other dementias in patients whose presentation is enigmatic, particularly early in the course of the illness, or in highly educated or intelligent individuals. The pattern of cognitive deficits may be suggestive of a specific disorder.

However, with all the tests that may be done, in some cases a diagnosis cannot be established for awhile, and the passage of time may be necessary to arrive at the proper conclusion. Specific biomarkers for the disease, possibly a panel of different tests, will probably be available in the near future to allow an earlier and more definitive resolution.

CLINICAL PICTURE

The major symptoms of Alzheimer's disease are noted in Table 3.2. Though impairment of short-term memory may be the most prominent symptom of Alzheimer's disease, all cognitive functions are eventually eroded. Episodic memory used to recall the information about our lives is involved early in the disease, since it is dependent on the hippocampus and medial temporal lobe. Semantic memory which entails knowing the names of objects and their function, and our general knowledge about the world, may be compromised next. But as the disease progresses, all aspects of memory deteriorate and patients may be unable to remember the names of their children or spouses, how old they are or where they

Table 3.2
Major Symptoms of Alzheimer's Disease

1) Memory impairment
2) Language dysfunction
3) Visual-spatial deficits
4) Impaired executive function
5) Behavioral disturbances

live. There is difficulty learning new information or tasks, and recalling things previously learned. Patients may ask the same questions repeatedly, forgetting the answers recently given.

Language dysfunction is also common in Alzheimer's, and it can be mild or quite severe, suggesting damage to the left hemisphere of the brain where language is based. This is called aphasia and may encompass all aspects of speech. There may be difficulty finding words and expressing one's self, or speech may be totally nonsensical with an inability to communicate needs. Understanding what is said may also be a problem and the Alzheimer's patient may be unable to follow complex or even simple instructions. Apraxia, or an inability to comprehend what a task entails and perform it, may also be seen. An interesting example of this is so-called dressing apraxia where an individual cannot put on a shirt or pants, because he or she cannot fathom where the arms and legs belong, or cannot recall the proper sequence of motor acts to perform the task. At times, agnosia may be found as well: difficulty recognizing a face, an object or a body part.

Visual spatial problems, which indicate right hemispheric impairment, occur frequently. This may be seen if the subject is asked to copy geometric figures or draw a clock. It may be responsible for curtailing daily activities because the person gets lost: a combination of visuo-spatial disorientation and memory dysfunction. When severe, it is even manifest within the home, where the person cannot find his or her way from room to room unaided.

Compromised executive function is inevitable in Alzheimer's patients at some point during their illness. Affected individuals cannot plan or organize activities, and are unable to pursue long-term or even short-term goals. They have trouble making decisions and lack the initiative to get things done, appearing unable to program the necessary steps to act on specific objectives. This may be part of the reason for the apathy in some of these patients. Loss of executive function constrains an individual in a tight box, where he or she is dependent on others to run his or her life. But generally, the person involved does not care and may not even be aware a problem exists.

Behavioral disturbances and changes in affect are also frequently a part of the picture, running the gamut from anxiety to depression, and from disinhibition to paranoia. As mentioned, depression may predispose a person to Alzheimer's or be integral to the disease process. It may be mild or severe, and may reflect an understanding on some level that something is wrong. Anxiety may coexist with depression or be free-standing, often arising out of unfamiliarity with a situation or place, or lack of comprehension about how to act or what to do. Disinhibition indicates a lack of social restraint shown by inappropriate behavior or speech. It is believed to result from damage to the frontal lobes of the brain. While more prominent in fronto-temporal dementia, it is common in Alzheimer's as well. Paranoid thinking and behavior are often seen as the disease progresses, with fantasies of a spouse being unfaithful or of people stealing. It may be related to the person's forgetfulness or lack of judgment and reasoning power. Delusions and hallucinations also occur, and wandering is not an infrequent problem.

Incontinence of stool and urine is common in the mid to latter stages of the disease. There may be multiple reasons why this happens, including forgetting to go to the bathroom until it's too late, not remembering how to get undressed, a lack of understanding about how and why it is necessary to use the bathroom, not knowing where the bathroom is located, social indifference, obeying primitive urges and simply an inability to control sphincters. The use of adult diapers may be required.

The final years of deterioration for the patient with Alzheimer's are particularly difficult for the families, with motor ability and balance increasingly impaired. Patients are eventually unable to walk and require wheelchairs, or become bedridden. Speech is totally unintelligible and there may be difficulty swallowing. Catheters may be placed to control urinary incontinence. Seizures may occur in some patients and twitches of the extremities or the whole body called myoclonic jerks may be seen. A point is reached where the patient may no longer be able to eat and may require a feeding tube for nutritional support. There is no resemblance to the loved one this person once was, and no communication or recognition emanates from his or her damaged brain. Death may come from pneumonia, possibly brought on by aspiration, as the individual is unable to handle secretions or fluids. Urinary tract infections also may cause the individual's demise, as can bed sores (decubitus ulcers) which may result in overwhelming infections. The usual duration of the disease is 5 to 8 years, but occasionally as rapid as 2 years, or drawn out over 15 to 20.

TREATMENT

Treatment falls into the categories of general measures that may be of value, psychiatric drugs to modify behavior, and medications specific for Alzheimer's. Some supportive measures may also be helpful (see Table 3.3).

Table 3.3
Current Treatment of Alzheimer's Disease

1) General measures
   a) Antioxidants
      Vitamin E, Selegiline, ginko biloba, "antioxidant cocktail"
   b) Anti-inflammatory drugs
      NSAIDs
   c) Aspirin
   d) Statins
   e) Blood pressure control
   f) Antidepressants
   g) Nutrition
   h) Exercise
   i) Cognitive intervention
2) Cholinesterase inhibitors
      Donepezil, galantamine, rivastigmine
3) Memantine
4) Psychiatric medications for behavioral disturbances
5) Supportive therapy

General Measures

Antioxidants

Free radicals generated by beta-amyloid 42 in Alzheimer's disease increase oxidative stress and appear to play a role in neuronal damage. Because of this, antioxidants have been used for some time both to prevent and treat Alzheimer's, but the benefits of specific compounds are in dispute. Vitamin E has antioxidative properties, theoretically neutralizing destructive free radicals, and is one of the substances that has been utilized. Past reports have shown it to be of possible value in delaying the progression of Alzheimer's patients to certain milestones of deterioration, and physicians have been prescribing it in doses as high as 2,000 IU daily. However, recent studies are ambiguous at best about its benefits and there is a suggestion that higher doses might actually be injurious to some patients. Thus, its use and the appropriate dosing remain uncertain. Other vitamins that are antioxidants such as vitamin D and vitamin C have been utilized as well, though not of proven worth in Alzheimer's. Some neurologists are also using "antioxidant cocktails," combining several different substances because of their theoretical effects rather than proven benefit. These cocktails may include vitamin E, vitamin C, acetyl-L-carnitine, alpha lipoic acid and coenzyme Q. (This will be discussed further in Chapter 11.)

A medication with antioxidant qualities called selegiline has also been employed to protect the brain in both Parkinson's disease and Alzheimer's, delaying progression of the diseases in some studies. The evidence for its utility is not clear cut.

Ginko biloba, a compound extracted from a plant of the same name, has been used for years by normal older people to enhance memory and brain function. It appears to act as an antioxidant and anti-inflammatory, with some anticoagulant properties as well, and has been given to some Alzheimer's patients though its efficacy is questionable.

Anti-inflammatory drugs

Since amyloid deposits in the brain cause inflammation that damages nerve cells and synapses, the use of anti-inflammatory medications has been tried both as a preventative and treatment. Non-steroidal drugs (NSAIDs) such as ibuprofen, naproxen and Cox-2 inhibitors (Vioxx and Celebrex) have been used for this purpose. A number of large studies did show some effect in terms of prevention, but there is no hard evidence that it is helpful in treating patients who already have Alzheimer's. However, since it is relatively benign and the disease is so devastating, some physicians have given NSAIDs in small doses as adjunctive therapy. (These will all be discussed in Chapter 11.) There is a possibility that another mechanism for NSAIDs may be at work in addition to their suppression of inflammation. Some of these compounds may reduce the activity of an enzyme called gamma-secretase that is responsible for breaking down amyloid precursor protein and generating beta-amyloid 42,[18] the substance believed most responsible for Alzheimer's.

Aspirin

Aspirin prophylaxis against heart attacks and strokes is probably worthwhile in any person above age 50 who does not have specific contraindications such as bleeding ulcers or aspirin allergy. Though it does not appear to significantly alter the Alzheimer's process in any way, its use in patients with this disorder is warranted to decrease cerebrovascular disease and small strokes which may heighten cognitive problems. A baby aspirin (81mg) is sufficient for this purpose. In addition to coating platelets in the blood and reducing clotting, it may have some mild anti-inflammatory effects on the blood vessels and possibly in the brain itself.

Statins

Statin drugs (Lipitor, Mevacor, Pravachol, Crestor), also known as HMG-CoA reductase inhibitors, have become widely used in our middle and older aged population because of their ability to lower lipids and cholesterol. They also augment endothelial cell function (the internal layer of the arteries), inhibit thrombosis (clotting) and reduce atherosclerotic vascular disease, heart attacks and strokes. In addition to the above actions, statins are known to have anti-inflammatory properties.[19] Though adverse effects do occur with these medications, they are relatively uncommon and usually reversible by stopping the drugs. Studies have been ambiguous as to the value of statins in preventing dementia and Alzheimer's disease,[20] with some showing positive results and others suggesting little benefit. But the use of statins in both treatment and prevention is believed to remain worthy of exploration, with larger trials necessary.

There are a number of reasons why statins may be of value in the prophylaxis and therapy of Alzheimer's. As mentioned previously, Alzheimer's and vascular disease of the brain often coexist. If diminished blood flow through the small arteries of the brain could be increased, or at least prevented from getting worse by arresting atherosclerosis, this might augment cognitive function in patients with dementia. Statins may have this type of effect. An increase in senile plaques and neurofibrillary tangles in patients with large vessel atherosclerotic disease has also been found.[21] Perhaps statins act here to impact Alzheimer's. Elevated cholesterol levels in the blood also seem to be associated with greater production of beta-amyloid 42 (the toxic form) by the brain. Since statins lower cholesterol in the blood, they may reduce beta-amyloid 42 in the brain as well. It is also believed by some investigators that statins may decrease the production of beta-amyloid 42 by shifting the pattern of breakdown of amyloid precursor protein (APP) by the brain enzymes (secretases) that do this. Or statins may lower phospho-tau in the brain. Statins might also work through their anti-inflammatory effect, eliminating some of the havoc amyloid wreaks on the brain. It is also possible statins combat Alzheimer's disease in a manner currently unknown.

There is one difference amongst statin drugs which should be taken into consideration. Some are able to penetrate into the brain through the blood-brain barrier because they are lipophilic (dissolve in fats), while others are not because they are hydrophilic (dissolve in water). Whatever mechanism or mechanisms can be evoked for statins in Alzheimer's disease, it appears there is enough suggestive evidence currently to use them in those patients with an elevated or borderline cholesterol level. But it has not yet reached a point where they should be employed universally in all people having the disease.

Blood pressure control

For some time, it has been recognized that hypertension increases the risk of dementia and Alzheimer's, though how that occurs is unclear. It may be simply that high blood pressure damages the small blood vessels and causes ischemic (diminished circulation) changes and mini-strokes in the white matter of the brain. The damage that takes place may be additive to that of the Alzheimer's process, and lowering the blood pressure may reduce the extent of any additional injury. There have been reports that a specific type of antihypertensive drug (brain penetrating ACE inhibitors) may be of particular value in patients with mild to moderate Alzheimer's disease and hypertension.[22] In addition to lowering blood pressure, these compounds may block the effects of excessive amounts of ACE (angiotensin-converting enzyme) in the hippocampus and frontal cortex of the brain in Alzheimer's patients, which may be playing a role in their cognitive decline.

Antidepressants

Antidepressants also have a role to play in the treatment of Alzheimer's, particularly early in the course when depression may be responsible for some of the symptoms. With the use of antidepressants, patients may be more alert, able to concentrate better, less apathetic and may actually show cognitive improvement. Of course, this does not last and as the disease worsens, these medications may no longer be helpful. The type of antidepressant utilized is important. The older group called tricyclics—amitriptyline, nortriptyline, doxepin, etc, may interfere with acetylcholine and make patients more confused. The newer kind of antidepressants called SSRIs (selective seratonin uptake inhibitors)—zoloft, celexa, lexapro—are the ones that should be employed when depression and dementia coexist.

Nutrition

Though Alzheimer's patients are able to obtain and prepare food for themselves in the early stages, adequate food intake soon falls into the province of the caregivers. While proper nutrition appears to reduce the chances of developing Alzheimer's, its role in treatment is less clear. Weight loss in older individuals has been felt to be a risk factor for Alzheimer's, or perhaps an early indication of the disease's presence. There has also been some evidence that continued weight loss in Alzheimer's patients is a predictor of more rapid cognitive decline. Reports from France seem to show that overall deterioration can be slowed by improved nutrition and weight gain in these patients. In a small study, Japanese investigators have demonstrated stabilization or even improvement of cognitive function over a 30-month period in Alzheimer's patients who adhered to a traditional Japanese diet high in fish and vegetables and avoiding meat and saturated fats.[23] Further evaluation is needed to assess the benefits of this approach.

Exercise

Exercise also appears to play a role in the prevention of Alzheimer's. When the disease is already present, exercise seems to improve the quality of life, enhancing mood and lessening behavioral disturbances. Whether it is beneficial in terms of cognitive deterioration is uncertain. However, recent animal data has shown positive effects of exercise in transgenic mice with Alzheimer's pathology.[24] A reduction of beta-amyloid deposits in the brain was correlated with the amount of running these mice did: the more activity, the less amyloid was found. The mechanism was unclear though several hypotheses were proposed. Exercise also appeared to be neuroprotective, with longer neuronal survival, neurogenesis and increased circulation to the brain. Whether these effects will be translatable to the human form of Alzheimer's disease remains to be seen after well-devised studies in large populations have been done.

Cognitive intervention

Cognitive therapy appears to help normal older people improve function and independent living,[25] and may be of some value in mild cognitive impairment, but the benefits are questionable in Alzheimer's patients. It is possible that in the initial phases, it may help affected people with the tasks of daily living and temporarily retard cognitive decline, but it does not appear to alter the disease process. The training uses cognitive abilities that are relatively intact to compensate for those that are lost, recognizing the humanity of these individuals. Quality of life may be improved and the patient's autonomy extended somewhat with this type of therapy.

A number of different programs have been created, and are being utilized and evaluated. The last word on these is not yet in.

There are two classes of drugs now being employed that appear to modulate some of the Alzheimer's effects in the brain, though not impacting the pathologic process. While these compounds are of some value, they are far from the answer to the problem of Alzheimer's disease.

Cholinesterase Inhibitors

Cholinesterase inhibitors began to be used for the treatment of Alzheimer's disease over 10 years ago, but the initial medication (tacrine) caused liver damage and was difficult to administer. The second generation of medications—Donepezil (Aricept), rivastigmine (Exelon) and galantamine (Reminyl, aka Razadyne)—have been much better tolerated and easier to give. They are currently felt by most neurologists to be the primary therapy for Alzheimer's,[26] though some believe the cost-benefit ratio does not warrant their extensive use. Recently there was a proposal to remove all medications employed to treat dementia from the formulary of the National Health System of Great Britain, indicating that they were not cost effective,[27] even though "the drugs provide moderate, short-term cognitive and behavioral benefit for some Alzheimer's patients."

The rationale for the drugs is straight forward. The neurotransmitter acetylcholine, which is critical in memory pathways and other cognitive functions, is diminished in patients with Alzheimer's disease. The cholinesterase inhibitors prevent the breakdown of acetylcholine in the synapses allowing more to be available to transmit impulses. Of course, this is dependent on the production of acetylcholine by intact neurons and its action on other intact neurons. As these cells die off with progression of the disease, the medications are of less value.

Used early in the course of the disease, patients may stabilize on the cholinesterase inhibitors and occasionally improve slightly, usually for a period of 6 to 12 months, though at times longer.[28] They may be more alert and better able to perform the tasks of daily living. Even after the cognitive decline resumes, there is a suggestion that these medications may help with behavioral symptoms, with patients on them being easier to manage, having less agitation and wandering.[29] Some studies also show that cholinesterase inhibitors decrease the time needed for caregiving and may delay the necessity of nursing home placement, allowing Alzheimer's patients to remain at home longer. If this is valid, it could represent significant savings to society and the families of these patients.

Besides cost, there are adverse effects from the cholinesterase inhibitors that need to be considered, and differences in dosing. The major impediment to their use are GI symptoms, particularly diarrhea and abdominal cramps, nausea and vomiting. Diminished appetite, fatigue and dizziness are also seen along with insomnia and muscle cramps. Donepezil may be somewhat better tolerated than the other two and is only taken only once a day, though a new form of galantamine is also once daily. There is only one step-up in dosing for Donepezil, while rivastigmine and galantamine have several increments in dosing. In demented patients who may rely on others for their medications, once a day dosing and less changes can mean better compliance. If a patient has side effects or no response to one cholinesterase inhibitor, it is probably worthwhile switching to another to see if the patient does better. There are also some secondary actions of galantamine and rivastigmine of possible benefit for Alzheimer's patients (nicotinic modulation and butyrl cholinesterase inhibition) in addition to its cholinesterase inhibition.

Memantine (Namenda)

Memantine's mechanism of action is quite different than the other medications currently being used. A chemical called glutamate in the brain is an excitatory neurotransmitter that may overstimulate certain receptors (NMDA or N-methyl-d-aspartate) in neurodegenerative disorders such as Alzheimer's, causing damage and possible cell death. Memantine theoretically blocks that effect and protects the neurons, as it is an NMDA antagonist. (NMDA receptors are believed to play a role in learning and memory.)

Studies have shown a reduction in clinical deterioration[30] in moderate to severe Alzheimer's patients on memantine and the FDA has given its approval for use in that group. It also appears to reduce the burden of the caregiver by making patients more compliant. Studies are ongoing in mild to moderate Alzheimer's patients and in MCI to show whether there is efficacy for memantine in these individuals. Some physicians are already utilizing it in these patients if they are unable to tolerate cholinesterase inhibitors, or if they are progressing while on them. Memantine can be used alone or in combination with cholinesterase inhibitors. Side effects are infrequent though transient confusion is occasionally seen. Unfortunately, this medication is also not a home run in the treatment of Alzheimer's, with temporary stabilization or incremental improvement the best that can be accomplished.

Psychiatric Medications

When patients with Alzheimer's disease are anxious, agitated or paranoid, it may be necessary to treat them with various tranquilizers to control their behavior, in addition to cholinesterase inhibitors and memantine. The medications employed depend on the prescribing physician's preference and the severity of the patient's problem. All of them have sedative effects and some of them can produce Parkinson's-like symptoms or abnormal movements called dyskinesias. But they may be required to deliver proper care and prevent the patient from injuring him or herself, or other people. Medications used include Risperdal, Zyprexa, Seroquel, Geodon and Abilify. Occasionally, minor tranquilizers such as lorazepam or aprazolam can be helpful as well. Before using aggressive drug therapy, caregiving issues or medical causes should be sought for behavioral problems, such as recurrent pain from any source that the patient can't describe. Environmental stresses including excessive heat or cold in the home, or loud noises which might produce agitation, should also be excluded.

Supportive Therapy

Supportive treatment to maintain Alzheimer's patients and preserve the best quality of life possible for them is quite important, considering that their judgment is impaired and there are many mundane tasks they are unable to perform for themselves. Exercise and nutrition have been mentioned and measures to ensure good hygiene should be observed. Socialization is also beneficial in those who are mildly to moderately affected, and situations that encourage this should be pursued: old friends, senior centers, Alzheimer's groups.

An early problem families have to resolve is the issue of driving, because removal of these privileges severely limits independence. Though even most mild Alzheimer's patients have some impairment when given on-road driving tests, they are usually able to drive locally,[31] when the routes are familiar. It is important however to err on the side of caution when the question arises of when a parent or spouse should stop driving, as it inevitably does. Other safety issues must also be addressed. At some point, a controlled environment may be required, perhaps locking the doors of the house to prevent wandering. Monitoring the use of the stove, especially gas, eliminating smoking of any sort, prohibiting power tools, are all measures that must be taken. Eventually, a need for 24-hour care arises when it is evident a person cannot live alone. Each family finds its own solution. Those affluent enough may hire a full-time companion to live with the patient. Or responsibilities may be shared by a spouse, children and a part-time caregiver. Or a child or spouse may assume total oversight. Community adult day care programs may also be helpful. But however it is done, the burden usually becomes too overwhelming in a home setting and the patient is transferred to a nursing home in the final stages.

FUTURE THERAPIES

As the disease process in Alzheimer's has been elucidated over the past two decades, methods of attacking it and points of attack have been theorized, leading to the two therapies now being used, experimental treatments being tried and new treatments that are on the drawing board (see Table 3.4). Since the preponderance of evidence suggests that soluble forms or deposits of beta-amyloid 42 in the brain are mainly responsible for the disruption of cell function and ultimately cell death, preventing amyloid generation, blocking its accumulation or getting rid of it once it has been produced seem to be the paths to pursue in order to control the disease.

The use of a vaccine to produce an immune response against beta-amyloid has received much attention in recent years, with a host of studies and articles about this approach.[32] Amyloid is a complex substance and the vaccines developed utilize a small fragment of the molecule which is injected in the hope that the body will produce antibodies (a protein that binds foreign proteins) against amyloid. These antibodies when attached

Table 3.4
Future and Experimental Therapies

1) Immune therapy
   a) Vaccines against amyloid or amyloid fragments
   b) Monoclonal antibodies
   c) IVIG
2) GAG mimetic drugs—Alzhemed
3) Substances that bind metal ions—Clinoquinol
4) Secretase inhibitors
5) Gene therapy
6) Reducing tau hyperphosphorylation
7) Stem cell therapy
8) Other therapies

to amyloid render it less toxic and allow the body's defenses to destroy this substance and remove it from the brain. This construct was found to work in transgenic mouse models of Alzheimer's where it did reduce the "amyloid burden," prevented new amyloid from forming, slowed inflammation and decreased the formation of abnormal nerve endings.

In a small study, a vaccine did produce a positive antibody response in some human subjects. However, many did not develop an immune response and a percentage of those who did also suffered meningoencephalitis[33] (inflammation of the brain and its covering) of immune origin. Though this reaction was detrimental, it may have happened because the vaccine was working against the amyloid deposits. There was also a suggestion that individuals receiving this treatment showed less cognitive decline than those who were untreated. And patients who died and were autopsied did show a significant reduction of amyloid plaques, indicating clearance of amyloid from brain tissue. The concept appears to have great promise and the challenge now is to find a vaccine that will target amyloid without damaging the brain. It may also be possible through genomic analysis techniques using gene expression patterns to determine before immunization which subjects are likely to develop meningoencephalitis and which are most likely to respond to this therapy.[34]

Most people have naturally occurring antibodies to amyloid in their blood, but Alzheimer's patients tend to have much lower levels than normal individuals. Another way to attack amyloid in the brains of Alzheimer's patients might be to use concentrated doses of antibodies from other people.[35] These antibodies can be found in human intravenous immunoglobulin (IVIG) collected from the blood of healthy donors. IVIG has been used to treat various illnesses for many years with a good safety record. The early results in a recent clinical trial where Alzheimer's patients were given IVIG was apparently encouraging, with cognitive decline being halted and some patients having improved. Hopefully, the preliminary results will be borne out when a larger study is done. However, this would not appear to be an answer to the riddle of Alzheimer's, as IVIG treatments are extraordinarily expensive, and enough IVIG to treat large numbers of patients could not be obtained.

Yet another immunologic approach to reducing amyloid in the brains of Alzheimer's patients is to employ "passive immunization": giving monoclonal antibodies that have been synthesized to act against amyloid or an amyloid fragment, bypassing the need for a human host response. With cell cultures and genetic engineering, large volumes of monoclonal antibodies against specific proteins can be generated. Using amyloid or one of its fragments to create the antibodies, a weapon can be produced that will attack amyloid. In transgenic mice with deposits of amyloid in their brains this model works, and initial clinical trials in humans have just begun. An intranasal vaccine has also been used successfully in mice. The question, of course, is whether the monoclonal antibodies will also cause meningoencephalitis in Alzheimer's patients as it clears amyloid from the brain. We will not know the answer until a number of patients have been treated.

A class of compounds called GAGs (glycosaminoglycans) in the brain binds to amyloid protein and enhances their conversion into fibrils and plaques which are toxic to neurons. Alzhemed, a new medication in Phase 2 trials, works by inhibiting the above process. It is called a GAG-mimetic drug because it mimics the actions of natural GAG and competes for the same binding site on amyloid protein, preventing the formation of amyloid fibrils. Alzhemed binds soluble beta-amyloid and promotes its clearance from the brain, reducing inflammation and toxicity. Though initial results are encouraging, it is too early to know whether it will become a significant therapeutic agent for Alzheimer's.

Various metal ions (copper, zinc, iron) appear to induce the deposition of amyloid in brain tissue and may also increase the oxidative damage caused by amyloid. A drug that was previously used to treat protozoan (one celled organisms) infections called clioquinol has been found to bind these metal ions and may have some value as a therapy for Alzheimer's. Though the drug can produce inflammation of the optic nerve, a small preliminary study showed improvement in Alzheimer's patients taking clioquinol without significant toxicity.[36] Larger trials are necessary to confirm efficacy and safety.

It was mentioned previously that amyloid precursor protein (APP), a very large molecule, is broken down by enzymes called secretases to form beta-amyloid 42. Both beta-secretase and gamma-secretase perform this function, and it has been shown that beta-secretase activity is increased in Alzheimer's patients in the areas of the brain where beta-amyloid is deposited.[37] Another enzyme, alpha-secretase, generates a type of amyloid that is less toxic to brain tissue. Research is ongoing to find substances that will block beta- and gamma-secretase and reduce the creation of beta-amyloid 42 in the brains of Alzheimer's patients. It appears that the active site of beta-secretase (also known as BACE-1) has been defined, allowing scientists to screen and modify compounds that will work at that site and inhibit the activity of beta-secretase. But there is a still a way to go before an effective drug will be available. However, a gamma-secretase inhibitor has recently been tested in 70 patients with apparently promising results.[38] Another possible method to reduce the amount of beta-amyloid 42 in Alzheimer's would be to channel the breakdown of APP to the alpha-secretase pathway, reducing the amount of beta-amyloid 42. Some investigators believe certain statin drugs may do this.

Gene therapy is another possible avenue being explored to treat Alzheimer's.[39] A gene utilized in a small group of patients controls the output of nerve growth factor (NGF), a protein that protects neurons from dying. In a small study, individuals given this appeared to show a slowing of cognitive decline. The patient's own skin cells in culture were infected with a virus that carried the gene into the cells, which then started producing nerve growth factor. These cells were subsequently injected into Alzheimer's patient's brains. Here, they were felt to work as biological pumps, sending NGF out into the tissues to stimulate regeneration of neurons. But it is too early to tell if this will really be a viable treatment option. Genes responsible for other substances that could theoretically halt the progression of Alzheimer's may be tried in the future.

A new class of anticholesterol drugs different from statins called ACAT inhibitors (acyl-coenzyme A: cholesterol acyltransferase) appears to be effective in blocking the creation of amyloid in transgenic mice. There was a dramatic reduction in amyloid deposition in the brains of these animals, learning appeared to be improved and the compounds were well tolerated. A decrease in soluble beta-amyloid in brain tissue was also noted. One of these compounds is in Phase III trials for cardiovascular disease and a study should be started soon in Alzheimer's patients.

Removing cerebrospinal fluid from the ventricular cavities of Alzheimer's patients and draining it into the peritoneal cavity through a plastic tube (ventricular-peritoneal shunt) has been suggested as a possible treatment for Alzheimer's. (It is currently used to treat normal pressure hydrocephalus which will be discussed later.) Though individuals with Alzheimer's were reported to have done better after this technique was used, most neurologists are skeptical. There does not appear to be any logical mechanism to explain why this should work, though the rationale is that shunting might mobilize amyloid and tau from the brains of Alzheimer's patients.

There have been reports that intravenous administration of insulin can improve memory in cognitively intact people or those with Alzheimer's disease. Whether this might lead to long standing benefits could not be tested, since repeated or prolonged use of IV insulin would cause low blood sugars and be dangerous. It has been found however that intranasal insulin is much safer and may be utilized more effectively by those areas of the brain responsible for memory,[40] though it seems to work better in Alzheimer's patients who do not carry the APOE 4 gene. Further evaluation of this therapy in a much larger group is necessary to determine the appropriate dosage, whether patients are truly improved, and whether it alters the course of the disease.

Substances that increase the activity of insulin degrading enzyme may also be useful in the future in treating Alzheimer's. This enzyme metabolizes beta-amyloid and inhibits the generation of the neurotoxic form, also blocking the aggregation of amyloid in senile plaques.

A compound called Flurizan (R-flurbiprofen) is currently in Phase 3 clinical trials in patients with Alzheimer's. An NSAID analogue, it appeared to be effective in tests on transgenic mice with an Alzheimer's-like condition. It is said to reduce both inflammation and levels of beta-amyloid 42, the latter effect possibly by modulating gamma-secretase activity in some way.

Another type of approach that does not target amyloid or inflammation in the brain is also being considered. Prevention of neurofibrillary tangles formed by hyperphosphoralated tau protein might limit the damage in Alzheimer's disease. (Amyloid appears to play a role in the creation of these neurofibrillary tangles.) Adding phosphorus to tau protein is believed to be a necessary step for this to occur within the cells, which is quite destructive to the microtubules. Certain enzymes called intracellular kinases are required for this to happen. Lithium (used to treat bi-polar illness) and divalproex (an epilepsy drug) inhibit the kinases. Thus, these drugs may be able to reduce hyperphosphoralated tau protein and neurofibrillary tangles, eliminating some of the cell death due to these tangles. Reinforcing the microtubules against the effects of phospho-tau and neurofibrillary tangles is also being tried with the use of an anticancer drug called taxol, thus far only in mice. However, if the neurofibrillary tangles are merely a by-product of the disease process rather than causative in some way, blocking their formation may not change the outcome.

Stem cell therapy has been touted in the media as a possible answer to the problem of Alzheimer's, but any type of useful treatment appears to be on the distant horizon if it is ever to happen. Stem cells are primitive cells derived from early embryos, umbilical cord blood, or bone marrow, that can theoretically develop into any type of cell depending on their environment and the stimuli they are given. It is hoped that if the proper stem cells are situated in the brains of patients with Alzheimer's, they will develop into neurons to replace those that have died off. However, there are many problems to be overcome before this possibility can become reality, including the fact that this therapy would not rid the brain of amyloid and its destructive effects.

A compound called xaliproden is also being tried in an experimental controlled study. It works specifically on nerve cells (neurotrophic) and appears to be neuroprotective, acting on damaged neurons and helping them recover function. Besides its direct effect, it may also stimulate the production of neurotrophic compounds by the brain to further enhance its benefits. Currently, we do not know whether or how successful it will be for the treatment of Alzheimer's.

In the future, the approach to the treatment of Alzheimer's may mirror current cancer chemotherapy, with a multipronged shotgun attack. We may see an Alzheimer's regimen that includes cholinesterase inhibitors, memantine or a similar drug, a particular NSAID that has an effect on the brain, a cocktail of antioxidant compounds, a substance similar to Clioquinol that binds metal ions and prevents the deposition of amyloid, and some type of antibody that directly attacks amyloid. Perhaps these can even be administered along with an exercise program and cognitive therapy. Of course, our ultimate goal is not to simply halt the progression of Alzheimer's once the disease process has started, but to prevent its occurrence.

Case History

Flora was a 64-year-old woman seen initially for neurologic evaluation in 1994 because of problems with memory. She had been born in Germany and had met her husband there 40 years earlier when he had been working as an investment banker, returning with him to the United States 2 years later. They lived on a small estate in an affluent neighboring town and she had never been employed. Her husband gave the history while she denied anything was wrong.

He noted that her problem had been present for about three years: minimal at first, but progressively worse. Recently, when he was out, Flora would call him many times during the day to ask him where he was. She had also begun to get confused while driving, but had not gotten lost yet. There had been difficulty understanding how to use the stove and dishwasher, even though he had gone over it with her many times. Not infrequently, when conversing, she could not remember what she had wanted to say. With a past history of depression, she had been started on small doses of Prozac by her internist. She had never had any significant medical illnesses, and was on hormone replacement therapy with estrace and provera. Throughout her life, she had been extremely religious and an avid church-goer, and obsessed about cleanliness, both personally and in her home. She had always exercised a great deal, walking or playing tennis most days.

Examination showed her to be fully oriented, but able to recall only one of three objects she had been told to remember after five minutes, and none of the three at ten minutes after they had been repeated for her. There was difficulty performing simple calculations, and she was unable to spell the word WORLD backward. Even though English was not her native tongue, there were no problems with language. She was told to take an aspirin and multiple vitamins daily, and various tests were ordered.

CT scan of her head showed some white matter changes in the brain interpreted as small vessel ischemic (decreased circulation) disease, with no other abnormalities. Blood tests were unremarkable. Formal neuro-psychological evaluation revealed global cognitive deficits with particu-larly severe impairment of memory and visuo-spatial skills. The picture was felt to be diagnostic of Alzheimer's.

Over the next two years, she progressed slowly and became more depressed, requiring higher doses of Prozac. She continued to walk daily with her husband and play tennis with friends, but was unable to keep score. Even local driving became impossible as she would get lost easily. In 1997, she was started on Donepezil when it became available. She developed headaches and it was stopped for a month, then restarted. In addition, she was told to take ibuprofen 400 mg twice a day and vitamin E 2,000 IU daily. With the institution of these medications, she seemed to be stable from a cognitive standpoint but became more obsessive about cleanliness, constantly scrubbing the floors and washing her hands. The Prozac was stopped and she was begun on Paxil with the hope it might calm her.

Over the next year, there appeared to be no progression. Her cholesterol was found to be slightly elevated and her internist prescribed Pravachol. At times when she was seen in the office, she seemed minimally better, being fully oriented and able to remember objects. But by the end of 1998, she was more irritable, angry and depressed, and was no longer able to cook meals. She was disoriented, could remember no objects she was instructed to remember, and had difficulty following commands, though there were still no language problems. Another antidepressant, Celexa, was tried but did not help with her agitation. During the next several months, she became increasingly anxious, had paranoid thoughts and followed her husband around the house. She refused to socialize with friends and was more confused. The Celexa was stopped and she was placed on Trazadone. The agitation improved slightly, but she continued to be reclusive and tracked every step of her husband's. In the months that followed, she began to have some stool incontinence, then urinary incontinence, and refused to go to daycare. She was also unable to dress herself.

Because of continued agitation, she was given Haldol, which made her sleepy and apathetic. She began having symptoms of Parkinson's disease (a side effect of Haldol) and was switched to Risperdal. There was no improvement in her agitation, but when her dose was increased she became apathetic again. More Parkinsonian signs also appeared. By 2001, she was babbling, irritable, completely disoriented, could not follow simple instructions and had difficulty feeding herself. She then began reciting Hail Marys incessantly, refused to change her clothes or listen to her husband, and manifested aggressive behavior. She was tried on Zyprexa and Seroquel, but remained irritable and combative. By early 2003, she had to be placed in a nursing home. Here, she began having myoclonic jerks (twitching of her extremities and whole body) and was started on Depakote, Welbutrin and Seroquel by a geriatric psychiatrist. Her speech became total gibberish and she was unable to walk. Wheelchair bound and in the nursing home, she is now apathetic with intermittent myoclonic jerks, no longer combative or agitated.

Case History

Joe was a 73-year-old man, a former high school history teacher with a doctorate in political science. He was first seen in 2002 because of a difficulty expressing himself which had started two to three years earlier and had slowly progressed. His memory had also deteriorated, particularly short-term. According to his wife, he was slow in processing information and had difficulty concentrating. There was no history of high blood pressure, heart disease, diabetes or strokes. He lived alone with his wife, who had also been a school teacher, in a small home in a nearby rural town.

On examination, he was fully oriented, knew who the president was and was able to spell WORLD backward. His speech was slightly hesitant but he could name objects well, repeat phrases and follow commands. There was difficulty with simple calculations, and he could recall none of three objects at five minutes, and none at ten minutes after reinforcement. The physical and neurological examination were otherwise normal aside from a blood pressure of 150/95 and a positive snout reflex (puckering of the lips when struck above—a primitive reflex seen with frontal lobe damage).

He was started on a baby aspirin, vitamin E 2,000 IU daily and folic acid, while his tests were pending. An MRI showed minimal white matter changes indicative of small vessel disease, and an EEG was normal. Formal neuropsychological testing revealed diminished ability to learn, major problems with memory, impaired language function, and problems with attention, processing speed and executive function. He was also noted to be slightly anxious. The diagnosis given was early dementia, most likely Alzheimer's.

When he returned to the office six weeks later, there was no change in his cognitive status and his blood pressure was still elevated. He had already been started on rivastigmine by his internist and was taking 3 mg twice daily. However, he was complaining of nausea, weight loss and poor appetite. The rivastigmine was stopped and he was advised to see his internist again to control his blood pressure and have his lipid profile and cholesterol checked. One week later, therapy was initiated with Donepezil. His cholesterol was subsequently found to be elevated and he was started on Lipitor.

Two months after beginning the Donepezil, his language function was the same, but his memory had improved slightly. For about 14 months, he remained stable. When he was thought to be somewhat worse, memantine was added to his regimen. Subsequently, slow progression of intellectual deficits were noted, with language ability and memory deteriorating. Over the past six months, his decline has accelerated. He has problems with immediate recall as well as short-term memory. There is difficulty dressing himself and he is unable to tell time. He has more problems expressing himself, naming things, repeating phrases and following commands. There are no behavioral problems and the remainder of his neurological examination is normal, with blood pressure and cholesterol controlled. His wife remains as his sole caregiver.

Case History

Katherine was a 79-year-old woman brought in by her husband. She had been seen initially for neurologic evaluation in August of 1997 because of memory problems, present for about a year and a half. She had retired from a job in retail sales 7 years earlier and lived with her husband in a small apartment. He reported that she misplaced things in the house, was unable to balance the checkbook, had stopped driving and did not do any shopping or cooking. She would also ask the same questions repeatedly. Aside from high blood pressure treated with medications, her medical and neurologic history were unremarkable. CT scan of the brain done prior to the consultation showed generalized atrophy, dilatation of the ventricles and small vessel disease.

Examination showed the patient to be disoriented to time and place. She did not know her address, had difficulty with calculations and could not spell WORLD backward. She could recall two of three objects at five minutes, then three of three at ten minutes. Her blood pressure was 170/90. Neurologic and physical examination were otherwise normal. Blood tests were ordered and her husband was told to start her on a baby aspirin, vitamin E and ibuprofen daily. She was to see her primary care doctor for blood pressure control and come back in six weeks.

However, she did not return until May of 1999. In the meantime, her primary care physician had started her on Donepezil 5 mg daily. She had continued her other medications and was also taking ginko biloba. Her husband reported that she had become more irritable, but he did not think her memory had changed. On testing, however, she was disoriented and could recall none of the three objects after five or ten minutes. She also had a positive snout reflex. Her Donepezil was increased to 10 mg daily and an MRI was ordered which revealed progression of the atrophy and small vessel disease.

Over the next several months, her memory became worse and she was more confused, though still able to dress and feed herself, and take care of hygiene. By September of 1999, she had become agitated and was unco-operative with any testing or examination. She was extremely suspicious and did not want to wait in the examining room while her condition was discussed with her husband. Her husband noted that he was having great difficulty getting her to take medications. Trazadone was prescribed to see if this would calm her.

During the following year, she became increasingly agitated, belliger-ent and neglectful of her own care. She was tried on various tranquilizers but refused to take any pills and her husband could not force her to do so. He brought in nurses and aides to help with her care, but she would not cooperate and was abusive toward them. Her behavior and cognitive function continued to deteriorate. By early 2001, she was frankly paranoid and combative. When seen in the office, she would not let her husband give any history, constantly interrupted him and would not allow herself to be examined. She denied anything was wrong with her. Her husband did not want to place her in a nursing home and was determined to care for her. Since she would not take any pills, she was started on Haldol solution which her husband managed to disguise in juices and foods. When seen toward the end of 2001, she was still paranoid and somewhat combative but less so and was more manageable at home. She still denied all symptoms, would not answer questions or be examined.

In January of 2002, it was noted that her agitation and combativeness were controlled. However, her balance was worse, with her walking slow and shuffling. She was cooperative with the examination but was disoriented, had difficulty performing simple tasks and had severely impaired short-term memory. The motor symptoms were felt to be due to the Haldol and her dosage was reduced.

Over the next year, she continued to decline, both cognitively and from a motor standpoint. The Haldol was switched to Risperdal. She became even more confused, unable to dress herself, could not follow or understand instructions. By the middle of 2002, she was walking with a slow, flexed posture and shuffling badly. She was sleeping most of the day, was incontinent and unable to do anything for herself. As she was no longer agitated, the Risperdal was reduced and then stopped, with little change. She no longer recognized her children nor asked about them, and needed assistance getting up from a chair. In September of 2002, she began falling at times and started having intermittent jerks. The following month, she had a generalized seizure and was hospitalized. From there she was transferred to a nursing home and was lost to follow-up.

Chapter 4

FRONTO-TEMPORAL DEMENTIA—PICK'S DISEASE

Everything that man esteems
Endures a moment or a day.

William Butler Yeats[1]

In 1892, the Czechoslovakian neurologist Dr. Arnold Pick described a form of dementia that was subsequently named after him. Pick's disease was different both clinically and pathologically from Alzheimer's which came to light more than a decade later. Yet for most of the twentieth century, Pick's and Alzheimer's diseases were lumped together as presenile dementias, rare conditions for which no treatment was available. Over the past three decades, however, the two illnesses have been differentiated from each other and are no longer considered rare. Pick's disease has also been placed under the umbrella of neurodegenerative disorders known as fronto-temporal dementias, because of the involved regions of the brain where the pathologic changes are most intense.

DEMOGRAPHICS AND GENETICS

Clinically, between 10 and 15 percent of individuals with dementia appear to fit the criteria for the condition known as fronto-temporal dementia (FTD). However, in autopsied cases of dementia, the percentage is far less and may actually be around 5 to 7 percent. Though originally it was believed that FTD/Pick's disease was a presenile dementia with the age of onset usually between 40 and 60, it is now known to affect all ages, with peak incidence between 55 and 65. Cases beginning after the age of 70 are uncommon. Unlike Alzheimer's, fronto-temporal dementia may occur with somewhat greater frequency among men than women, though many reports note no sexual predisposition.

There is a strong genetic component to fronto-temporal dementia, with 40 to 50 percent of those afflicted having a family member with the disease. The remainder of the cases are sporadic with no known genetic connection. Familial cases are passed down in an autosomal dominant pattern, a child of an affected parent having a 50 percent chance of acquiring the disease. A mutation of the tau gene on chromosome 17 may be responsible for about 15 percent of the hereditary cases. There have also been reports of abnormalities on chromosome 9 and chromosome 3. In some families with fronto-temporal dementia, ALS (Lou Gehrig's disease), Parkinsonism and psychiatric illnesses have been noted.

PATHOLOGICAL FEATURES

At autopsy there is atrophy of the frontal and anterior temporal lobes disproportionate to the remainder of the brain, though generalized atrophy may eventually occur. Unlike Alzheimer's, there is sparing of the hippocampus. Microscopically, one sees aggregates of abnormal tau protein in tangles within the nerve cells. Tau plays a vital role in maintaining cellular structure and microtubules, which are involved with transport of nutrients and other substances. The abnormal tau tangles disrupt cell function and eventually result in neuronal death, particularly of the larger neurons. This is most prominent in the anterior temporal and frontal lobes. A type of scarring unique to the central nervous system known as gliosis is seen as well, along with small holes in the cortex of the brain called vacuolation. In the Pick's form of FTD, Pick cells, which are ballooned achromatic (pale) neurons, are found along with inclusion bodies within the cells called Pick bodies, highlighted by special silver stains.

Fronto-temporal dementia falls into the category of neurodegenerative diseases known as tauopathies which are characterized by abnormalities of tau protein and aggregation into filaments. Other diseases in this grouping include progressive supranuclear palsy, corticobasal degeneration and motor neuron disease (amyotrophic lateral sclerosis—ALS). In the tauopathies there is an increase in the phosphorylation (addition of phosphorous) to tau protein, causing it to form filaments and tangles. A transgenic mouse model of tau dysfunction has been developed, which may help unravel the mechanisms of these diseases and lead to effective treatments. However, not all patients with FTD have abnormalities of the tau gene or protein.

Recent mouse studies have suggested that mutant tau protein which is toxic to neurons causes the damage in fronto-temporal dementia rather than the neurofibrillary tangles.[2] The neurofibrillary tangles do not correlate with, and are not responsible for, cognitive dysfunction or neuronal death, and may be protective in some way, or an incidental marker. By stopping the formation of the mutant tau protein, or encouraging its destruction and removal from the brain, we may be able to arrest the process, and according to this report, even reverse it.

DIAGNOSTIC EVALUATION

As with Alzheimer's disease, there are no specific tests or biomarkers that will lead to a definitive diagnosis. But the clinical picture, along with supporting laboratory data (particularly imaging), can forge a presumptive diagnosis with some degree of accuracy in most cases. However, a significant number of patients labeled as fronto-temporal dementia clinically are found to have Alzheimer's at postmortem, and vice versa.

The usual blood tests used to evaluate patients with dementia should be obtained, but will not be helpful. Lumbar puncture and spinal fluid evaluation will also not yield results favoring FTD, but should be done to exclude other less common causes of dementia.

CT scan or MRI may show a pattern of anterior temporal and frontal lobe atrophy, though sometimes this is not seen until the late stages. These tests also exclude slow growing brain tumors involving the frontal or temporal lobes which may present in a similar fashion to FTD. In patients with non-diagnostic imaging, functional MRI testing (fMRI) has been found to differentiate between fronto-temporal dementia and Alzheimer's.[3] However, while this test may be valuable in experimental studies, it is probably too complex for clinical practice.

PET scanning (positron emission tomography), using radioactive glucose as a marker, shows a decrease in metabolic activity in the frontal and temporal lobes. If the diagnosis remains questionable, a PET scan with C-PIB, which binds to amyloid, will establish whether or not the patient has Alzheimer's, which provides the most confusion with fronto-temporal dementia. However, at the moment, this type of PET scan is not widely available. SPECT scanning (single photon emission tomography) can also aid in diagnosis by showing diminished perfusion of blood in the frontal and temporal lobes.

Neuropsychological testing does not paint the typical picture expected in dementia, with memory ability remaining fairly intact until the disease is advanced. Indeed, MMSE testing may be completely normal when patients are first seen. More robust evaluations however, may show language difficulties, loss of social restraints and diminished executive function. All of these findings are noted in Alzheimer's as well, but usually in conjunction with considerable memory impairment. The above deficits without memory loss point to a diagnosis of fronto-temporal dementia.

CLINICAL PICTURE

Fronto-temporal dementia is a heterogeneous disorder both in terms of clinical presentation and pathology. As in most degenerative processes involving the brain, the onset of the disease is insidious, with family members often uncertain when it actually started. At times, a specific incident may make them aware that something is wrong, or language problems may become more obvious. Progression of the disease is generally slow, the entire course, from diagnosis to death, usually running 6 to 10 years. There are felt to be two major clinical subdivisions of fronto-temporal dementia, the frontal lobe variant and the temporal lobe variant, but there may be considerable overlap in symptoms.[4]

Frontal Lobe Variant

In the frontal lobe variant of the disease, behavioral abnormalities predominate, with changes in personality and social conduct. (Some investigators have found that behavioral abnormalities in fronto-temporal dementia are associated with right hemispheric atrophy.[5]) An MMSE or other standard tests that measure cognitive decline may reveal no alterations of function for some time. Memory in particular may be quite intact during the early stages. Occasionally, these patients may present to psychiatrists with behavioral changes that seem to suggest psychiatric illness, or even to the police for what looks like criminal actions. People with this condition generally have little insight that something is wrong and are not responsive to guidance from friends or family to change their behavior.

Virtually all of these patients have some degree of disinhibition and loss of social restraints, varying from mild to severe. They may show poor impulse control, doing or saying things that are inappropriate. Impatience or rudeness is common, with refusal to wait for one's turn when it is expected. Food may be grabbed and eaten immediately, with hands wiped on clothes or the furniture. Foul language may be used in situations where it is uncalled for, or wisecracks made about things that are not funny. Sometimes, speech may be abusive or things may be said that are embarrassing to friends or even strangers. Someone may be called fat or ugly, or their looks or clothing derided. Other people may be interrupted when they are speaking if the person with FTD has something to say, with a total lack of consideration.

Inappropriate and antisocial behavior may include taking things from friends or acquaintances, frank stealing or shoplifting. If caught, they may not be able to offer an explanation for what they have done. Aggressiveness and belligerency may occur in some cases, with the person starting verbal or physical brawls over minor slights or nothing at all. Sexual deviancy may also be seen, running the gamut from a man making inappropriate advances, exposing himself, masturbating in public or groping women, though rape or child molestation appear uncommon. Women may also manifest unexpected sexual behavior, acting seductively, dressing provocatively or making remarks that are out of place. People with this form of FTD show lack of concern about their behavior and its effects on family and friends. Indeed, these individuals may alienate those who are close to them with their speech and actions, to the point where they are abandoned and alone, or left with a spouse who is frustrated and angry.

Many of these patients are disinterested in their appearance and hygiene. Early on, they may dress inappropriately, such as wearing jeans and a sport shirt to a dinner party that requires a jacket and tie. Or they may wear outfits that don't match, in terms of color coordination, seasonality or level of formality. It may progress to the point where they are dressing in dirty or stained clothes, or torn clothes, or using the same outfits over and over again. They may not wash regularly or brush their teeth, or clean their nails, and may avoid taking showers or bath. A spouse or caregiver may have difficulty getting them to wash or wear clean clothes, as they are not distressed by what others may think and not motivated by any self-imposed standards.

Financial recklessness can also be seen at times. Money may be spent on items of little value, or things not needed, with savings squandered or debt increased without a second thought. Foolish investments may be made as well, as the affected person may not understand the ramifications of what he or she is doing, or may believe that a stock or business is going to soar, when it is more likely to plummet. Gambling is another way huge sums of money may be lost, with little remorse for the resources that were dissipated.

Ritualized and compulsive behavior also occurs in some of these men and women. This may include pacing back and forth and any type of stereotyped or repetitive movements or action. At times, frequent hand washing or placement of objects in certain patterns may be seen. There is great variability in behavior even by the same affected person, and so what is noted at one stage of the disease may not be present in another, or may be altered in form.

Though some individuals with the frontal variant of FTD may be disinhibited, saying whatever is on their minds and acting without restraint, others with this condition become apathetic and withdrawn. Instead of interactions with people that may be inappropriate and cause distress, they may shun social contact and become reclusive. They may be content to sit around all day without specific activities, perhaps watching television, playing solitaire or doing nothing. There may be a lack of spontaneity and imagination, and a rigidity in terms of what they do in their daily lives.

Impaired executive function may be prominent as well in some of these patients, contributing to their lack of activities. They have great difficulty or inability to plan any significant undertaking or organize their lives in any productive fashion. There appears to be a lack of initiative that may be projected as an unwillingness to do anything, but is really an inability to move from Step A to Step B. These people are unable to work at any job, and if they had been employed, they are invariably fired. Though this disturbance in executive function may be considered as laziness by observers, it is beyond the person's control and they cannot be prodded or motivated to change. This can be very frustrating for spouses, children or friends of the affected person.

Some individuals with this condition may manifest an increase in appetite, with constant eating and resultant weight gain. A desire for particular foods can be seen, frequently sweets, with the same thing being eaten again and again. In addition to changes in appetite, other normal physiologic drives, such as sleep and libido, may also be disrupted. There may also be an oral fixation in the advanced stages of the disease, with patients putting objects as well as food into their mouths. Excessive imbibing of alcohol can be another distressing symptom.

Though memory may be involved early in the course of the illness, it is not impacted to any major degree until later on. But as the disease progresses, memory and all other areas of cognitive functioning are compromised. Indeed, a point may be reached where a patient with fronto-temporal dementia and one with Alzheimer's can not be differentiated clinically.

Depression may also be present at the onset, occasionally masking some of the other symptoms.

Temporal Lobe Variant

In this form of fronto-temporal dementia, which is less common than the frontal variant, language function and speech are affected, particularly when the left temporal lobe is involved, with behavioral manifestations less prominent.[6] The temporal lobe variant is also called primary progressive aphasia, because of the problems that occur with language. Semantic dementia is another term utilized, but some question its validity because impaired recognition of objects and faces may not be present.[7] Primary progressive aphasia has been characterized as "a relentless dissolution of language with memory relatively preserved."[8] Often, the initial symptoms in the temporal lobe variant may be difficulty in finding words, or a hesitancy in speech. Problems naming objects (anomia) may also be seen. Patients usually have difficulty expressing themselves as well as understanding what has been said. Reading and writing are inevitably impaired at some point.

Sometimes, only nonsensical phrases are spoken, or even complete gibberish. Words or phrases may be repeated over and over. At times, the motor control of speech may also be deficient, with thickness or slurring of words known as dysarthria. In most cases, verbal output is progressively reduced, with spontaneous speech increasingly sparse. Eventually, affected individuals become mute. Memory again is relatively spared until the advanced phases. Visuo-spatial functions, which are often compromised early in Alzheimer's, seem to remain fairly intact in both forms of fronto-temporal dementia. During the initial stages of the disease, those people who do not depend on verbal ability for their livelihoods, such as manual laborers, masons, landscapers, etc, may be able to continue working as long as they are able to understand instructions. Ultimately, however, this is no longer feasible. Just as in Alzheimer's disease, problems with daily living occur in primary progressive aphasia, but it is because of language dysfunction rather than memory. While some patients with the temporal variant continue to have mainly language and speech problems as the disease evolves, others eventually develop behavioral disturbances, memory impairment and generalized cognitive decline.

In contrast to Alzheimer's, incontinence may be seen fairly early in a proportion of patients with either form of FTD. Disturbances of attention are noted as well, with inability to sustain a line of thought or continue a conversation. Patients may be easily distracted for any tasks. Over time, the clinical pictures of the frontal and temporal lobe variants may merge, and they may not be easily distinguishable. Motor symptoms may also occur, usually late in the course, with balance problems, stiffness in walking and incoordination. In addition, a small subgroup of patients with fronto-temporal dementia may develop motor neuron disease (ALS, Lou Gehrig's disease) or other conditions that are similar to Parkinson's disease. When the last stages of FTD are reached, swallowing may become difficult and patients may aspirate food. A superimposed infection such as pneumonia is often responsible for death.

TREATMENT

Unfortunately, there is no effective treatment for fronto-temporal dementia. The best that can be done is to try and alleviate symptoms and modify behavior, and even here, success is modest at best. Psychotherapy has not been shown to be of any value, as patients have no insight into their behavioral problems and no motivation to change. However, supportive care by understanding caregivers can be helpful at times. Control over finances should be taken away from the patient early and driving restricted. Any critical situation requiring judgement should be circumvented. Confronting obsessional behavior or inappropriate actions should be avoided, as it may lead to belligerent verbal or even physical responses. People with FTD should be coaxed gently to alter their behavior, recognizing that any change will likely be temporary, and the same process will soon have to be repeated.

Art therapy may be a way to modify the behavior of some of these patients. Painting, drawing, sculpting or pottery sometimes holds the interest of an individual with fronto-temporal dementia and allows him or her to work in a creative fashion while transiently overcoming aggressive or antisocial urges. It has been shown that some patients with FTD, particularly those with semantic dementia, become engrossed in painting and quite productive from an artistic standpoint, even as the disease progresses.[9] As mentioned previously, the visuo-spatial deficits so common in Alzheimer's are rare in fronto-temporal dementia, imposing no limitations on artistic skills. Some of the inhibitions dominant in the personality of the person when he or she was "normal" may be overwhelmed by the disease process, eliminating any constrictions and unleashing that individual's innate creativity. Painting or drawing may utilize an obsessive style, with final products that are surrealistic or hyper-realistic, many fitting into the category of what could be called "outsider art."

Speech therapy and occupational therapy may occasionally be of benefit, and jigsaw puzzles and electronic games may be worthwhile for some patients. In addition, regular exercise, such as brisk walking, should be encouraged. A social worker or case manager should be engaged early to help with management issues, making the condition more tolerable for the patient and family. Counseling, speech therapy and cognitive therapy may also be of some limited help.

Making an accurate diagnosis can guide the use of medications. Cholinesterase inhibitors employed for Alzheimer's patients have not been shown to benefit those with fronto-temporal dementia and there have been some reports that they may increase aggressive behavior. As yet, there is also no evidence memantine is helpful. That being said, a brief course of one or both of these may be tried under careful observation, because there is no definitive therapy available and an occasional patient might respond. SSRIs (selective serotonin re-uptake inhibitors) may be of some value in alleviating symptoms of depression, and also of help to those with behavioral disturbances. Stimulants such as amphetamines and Ritalin have also been used in individuals with the frontal lobe variant and dysfunctional conduct, attentional problems or depression, but with no data supporting their effectiveness. Trazadone has been given if there is difficulty sleeping, and the atypical antipsychotic drugs have been utilized when behavioral abnormalities are unmanageable. The bottom line, of course, is that we are treating symptoms and doing nothing to alter the disease itself. But with the pathologic process responsible for FTD being better understood and new work going on to further delineate the causitive mechanisms, perhaps effective therapy will be available in the near future.

Case History

Philip, a 67-year-old man, was first seen by a neurologist in September of 1996. He was accompanied by his wife who complained that he was having difficulty with memory and concentration, and had some confusion. The patient denied there were any problems. He had a Bachelor's and Master's Degree in Chemistry, and had taught at a local community college before retiring three years earlier. There was a history of excessive alcohol intake and prior hypertension. His mother had been diagnosed as having dementia, but the circumstances and diagnosis were unclear. Neurologic examination was completely normal as was blood pressure, and he scored 29/30 on MMSE.

The patient was referred to a neuropsychologist for formal testing the following month and she made a diagnosis of Alzheimer's after a full battery of tests. These showed minor problems with executive function, impulsivity, concrete thinking, impaired problem solving and attention, with some difficulty naming and minimal impairment of memory. However, in her report, the examiner noted the wife's description of the patient as being socially inappropriate, his constant use of "bathroom humor" and her frustration at his inactivity, lack of initiative and motivation. The examiner also commented on the patient's quips being sexist and inappropriate, and repeating stories he had told in previous sessions.

MRI of the brain and EEG were reported as normal and various blood tests were unremarkable. When the patient was seen by the neurologist a month later, he was started on selegiline 5 mg twice a day, vitamin E 400 mg twice a day, and aspirin. His next visit was in March of 1997 and Aricept 5 mg daily was begun. The following visit, his wife thought his memory had slightly improved. The Aricept was subsequently increased to 10 mg daily.

Through the remainder of 1997 and early 1998, Philip was apparently unchanged, but by August of 1998, his wife reported increasingly inappropriate speech and behavior. There were verbal outbursts of temper and he had become more rigid regarding his schedule, with agitation when his routine was disrupted. He was still driving locally at this time. In December of 1998, his wife noted that he could not travel with her in groups because of his offensive language. Follow-up neuropsychological testing at that time showed his memory still fairly intact, but inappropriate jocularity during the interview. The other parameters were minimally worse.

During 1999 and 2000, he became progressively disinhibited, with frequent crude comments. He was also more slovenly in his dress. His memory ability and language function did not change appreciably. Indeed, his MMSE was 28/30 in October of 2000. His wife noted at that time that he was no longer showering and that they argued when she urged him to wash himself.

Over the next year, he was essentially stable, but his wife continued with the same complaints. In July of 2001, his MMSE was 27/30, but he was felt to be depressed and started on Paxil 10 mg daily. This did not seem to help him and was stopped. In October of 2001, his MMSE was the same and there were no differences in cognition or behavior. He continued to deny that anything was wrong. In March of 2002, the patient was sent for neuropsychological evaluation with a new examiner. On this exam, he was found to have significant deficits in language skills, including fluency and naming, and executive function. There were minor problems with immediate memory and attention. Visuo-spatial and sensory perception skills were intact. The examiner remarked that memory had declined little since the original testing five years earlier. Some degree of depression was also noted. Outside of formal testing, the patient's behavior was described as grossly inappropriate. There was also little insight or empathy into his actions when he was given feedback. The examiner thought that Philip had a progressive dementia, and for the first time, fronto-temporal dementia was mentioned as the likely cause.

Philip was seen by me initially in July of 2002. His wife declared that nothing had changed since his last visit to the other neurologist though his Aricept had been stopped and he had been switched to Exelon 3 mg twice a day. Other medications were the same. He was still driving and not getting lost, but following instructions was more difficult, he was insulting other people, was verbally abusive and hostile. On examination, he was fully oriented, and scored 27/30 on the MMSE. There were no other neurologic findings and his medications were continued. By October, however, his wife felt he was worse. He was confused at times, had more difficulty with directions and continued to be socially inappropriate. His Exelon was increased to 4.5 mg twice daily and when seen in November, his wife said he had improved slightly. He was having some diarrhea and abdominal cramps, so his Exelon dosage was not raised further. A repeat MRI of the brain was ordered which showed diffuse cerebral atrophy and some small vessel disease.

In January of 2003, his wife commented that he had deteriorated further. He was fully oriented and his MMSE was 25. Since he was no longer having diarrhea or cramps, Exelon was increased to 6 mg twice a day. When seen again in March, his wife felt he was better, being more animated and with improved memory. There was no change on testing and he was again very jocular and inappropriate.

Subsequently, the patient slowly declined. He was still driving locally in July of 2003 when he had a minor accident and driving was stopped. His blood pressure was found to be slightly elevated and his internist started him on Norvasc 5 mg daily. Some agitation was also occurring and problems with hygiene continued. Paxil 10 mg daily was again added to his regimen. By September, he was worse. His wife described him as childish and silly, bothering her and anyone who was around. The Paxil was stopped. In December, his wife said that he spent all day sitting and watching television and had no initiative at all. He was still refusing to bathe and was getting up in the middle of the night and pacing about.

At the end of January 2004, he began having frequent myoclonic jerks (sudden jerks of his extremities or body). With a negative EEG, he was started on depakote (an anticonvulsant) 250 mg at bedtime which controlled the movements. In May of 2004, he had a brief generalized seizure and the depakote was increased to twice daily. EEG was again negative. He continued to get progressively worse over the next year and a half, becoming disoriented to time and place, and with impaired short-term memory. By May of 2005, he began to have difficulty with walking and balance, and was increasingly confused. He remained inappropriate with his comments and was still making off color jokes. When seen in August, he was apathetic with little spontaneous speech.

Chapter 5

DEMENTIA WITH LEWY BODIES AND PARKINSON'S DISEASE DEMENTIA

In old age the activity of the mind . . . declines only through the decay of some other inward part.

Aristotle—On The Soul[1]

Plan for the difficult while it is easy.

Te Tao Ching[2]

The above two conditions are considered together in this chapter because the disease processes are similar, though different parts of the brain are predominantly affected by each entity. Lewy bodies are present in the neurons in both illnesses and the clinical pictures include the motor findings of Parkinson's disease and cognitive decline. However, in Dementia with Lewy bodies (DLB), intellectual impairment is evident initially, or soon afterward, whereas in Parkinson's disease dementia (PDD) occurs later on. Under previous criteria "if the dementia was present within one year of the onset of motor symptoms, the individual had DLB, otherwise it was Parkinson's disease dementia." A recent conference declared that using a "one year rule" to make a diagnosis of DLB was too arbitrary, and the presence of dementia at onset of symptoms was felt to be the defining characteristic of the condition.[3] But this also appears to be arbitrary, and it may be wrong to separate what may be one disease into two on the basis of when particular symptoms make their appearance. Nevertheless, in this chapter we will describe Dementia with Lewy bodies and Parkinson's disease dementia as two distinct disorders.

Besides the overlap of DLB and Parkinson's disease dementia clinically and pathologically, both conditions also share attributes with Alzheimer's, which often coexists in the same person, creating a spectrum of diseases whose bands are interwoven. At times, it may be impossible to identify which symptoms of dysfunction in an affected individual are being caused by which processes. The possible relationships among Parkinson's disease, DLB and Alzheimer's, are as follows:

Parkinson's disease <> DLB <> Lewy body variant of Alzheimer's <> Alzheimer's disease

DEMENTIA WITH LEWY BODIES

In 1912, Dr. Frederich Heinrich Lewy, a contemporary of Dr. Alois Alzheimer, described neuronal inclusion bodies in the brains of patients with Parkinson's disease. Subsequently, these abnormal protein deposits were named after him. In his cases and later pathologic studies of Parkinson's disease, Lewy bodies were found in the deep gray matter of the brain. It was not until the 1960s that Lewy bodies were also noted in the cells of the cortex in some demented patients. This was considered to be a rare finding until the mid-1980s, when new and more sensitive staining techniques discovered Lewy bodies to be quite common in individuals with dementia. By 1995, Dementia with Lewy bodies became accepted terminology for patients with a variety of clinical syndromes, all of whom had similar pathology in the brain.

DEMOGRAPHICS AND GENETICS

Thus far, no genetic pattern for dementia with Lewy bodies has been elucidated, though there have been multiple cases in some families. A recent study proposes that mutations in the beta-synuclein gene may predispose individuals to the development of dementia with Lewy bodies, but further investigation of this is required.[4] The presence of the APOE 4 genotype may be increased in patients with DLB, but only in those who also have Alzheimer's pathology. No predilection for the disease has been found in any particular racial group. There is a suggestion that DLB may occur slightly more frequently in men than women, but no specific risk factors have yet been uncovered.

The statistics on the incidence and prevalence of Dementia with Lewy bodies are confusing. The usual figures have DLB responsible for 10–20 percent of all cases of dementia, though there have been claims it is higher or lower. Some reports have it as the second most common cause of dementia after Alzheimer's,[5] though that raises the question of where vascular dementia fits in. Part of the problem is defining DLB itself. In the medical literature, dementia with Lewy bodies has been described with a number of different names, all refering to the same condition. And there are other questions that further muddy the waters. Are those patients with Parkinson's who develop dementia part of the group, or a separate condition? Into what category does a person with both the pathologic changes of Alzheimer's and DLB fit? There are so many combinations and overlaps both clinically and pathologically that it is hard to arrive at any conclusions about the frequency of DLB. Of course, that is also true about vascular dementia, where there may be concurrent changes of Alzheimer's and/or Lewy body disease.

DLB tends to come on somewhat more abruptly than Alzheimer's and may have a more rapidly progressive course, generally lasting from 5 to 7 years. Caring for patients with DLB costs considerably more annually than those with Alzheimer's disease.[6] The psychiatric manifestations and the Parkinsonian components appear to be responsible for the difference.

PATHOLOGICAL FEATURES

We will describe the pathology of DLB and PDD separately, acknowledging the similarity in findings and realizing that in the future they may be categorized as one entity. At autopsy, the brains of patients with DLB may appear normal, though diffuse atrophy can be present with shrinkage of the cerebral cortex. Microscopically, the hallmark of the disease is the Lewy body. This is a spherical inclusion within cells that has a dense hyaline core, surrounded by a clear halo. Lewy bodies consist of a proteinaceous material that includes alpha-synuclein (a pre-synaptic protein), neurofilament proteins and another protein called ubiquitin. Special stains for ubiquitin or alpha-synuclein highlight the Lewy bodies. They are found in both the deep structures of the brain and cerebral cortex, but in DLB are more prominent in the cortex and limbic system (the brain nuclei involved with emotion), while in Parkinson's disease they are seen more in the deep gray matter. Far advanced cases of dementia with Lewy bodies and Parkinson's disease with dementia may look the same pathologically.

Abnormal neurites (projections from the neuronal cell body) are noted in DLB in the hippocampus and other areas of the brain, and are labeled as

Lewy neurites. Neurotransmitters in the brain are reduced, particularly dopamine and acetylcholine. Widespread death of cortical neurons, often present in Alzheimer's, does not occur. The clinical symptoms are probably related to the loss of neurotransmitters and interference with synaptic function. There is disruption of information flow and processing due to impairment of various neuronal circuits, particularly from the deep structures of the brain to the cortex of the frontal lobe. Occasionally, vacuolization (holes) are found in various regions. The pathologic changes of Alzheimer's, amyloid plaques and neurofibrillary tangles, may coexist with those of DLB in 30–50 percent of cases. To date, there is no coherent theory to explain the cause of dementia with Lewy bodies.

DIAGNOSTIC EVALUATION

The history, interview and physical examination may allow the clinician to make a presumptive diagnosis (see Table 5.1). Fluctuation in cognition, visual hallucinations and Parkinsonian signs are the signal features of the disease, and at least two of these three attributes must be present along with dementia. However, all three may also be seen in Parkinson's disease with dementia. As mentioned in the criteria used to distinguish the two conditions, patients with DLB must have cognitive impairment present from the beginning, while in Parkinson's it develops later. But confounding the clinical picture is the frequency of Alzheimer's coexisting with the other two entities.

The usual studies done in evaluating patients with dementia should be performed when DLB is suspected, mainly to exclude other conditions. This includes routine blood work, MRI and neuropsychological testing. A recent study found the volume of the putamen (one of the deep nuclei of the brain) diminished on MRI, indicating that it was atrophied.[7] This was not noted in individuals with Alzheimer's.

EEG and spinal tap are generally not helpful. Diagnosis may be aided by SPECT and PET scans which show decreased perfusion and metabolism in the occipital regions of the brain. The use of special radioactive

Table 5.1
Diagnosis of Dementia with Lewy Bodies

1) Fluctuation in cognitive ability with variation in attention and alertness
2) Recurrent visual hallucinations
3) Motor features of Parkinson's disease

markers reveals reduced activity in cells utilizing dopamine as a neurotransmitter in the deep nuclei of the brain.

Neuropsychological testing may also be of value. Significant visuo-perceptual and visuo-spatial problems together with relatively mild memory impairment makes dementia with Lewy bodies much more likely than Alzheimer's.[8] In addition to the differences in memory, patients with DLB have much more severe executive dysfunction than those with Alzheimer's disease on neuropsychological evaluation.[9]

CLINICAL PICTURE

Dementia with Lewy bodies generally follows a downhill course, with worsening cognitive impairment and the motor privations of Parkinson's disease. The intellectual deficits are those seen in all forms of dementia, with no specific pattern favoring DLB. Fluctuating levels of cognitive ability, alertness and attention, are however characteristic of this condition. The variability in symptoms may encompass time spans as short as moments, or as long as weeks. Patients may become suddenly confused or disoriented, not knowing where they are, the date or time. They may also have language problems, with trouble finding words or understanding a conversation, or with disorganized speech. At times, they may even be mute, yet appear to converse normally a few hours later. Also seen may be excessive daytime sleepiness and periods when the affected individual stares into space. This fluctuation in the patient's cognitive status can differentiate individuals with DLB from Alzheimer's and normal aging.[10]

Visual hallucinations, which are unusual in other types of dementia, are almost always present in DLB, with the patient often willing to describe what he or she is seeing: people, animals or inanimate objects. They are often not bothersome to that individual, and he or she may accept their presence without anxiety, understanding that they are imaginary. Less frequent are auditory hallucinations, or those involving smell or taste. Delusions may also occur on occasion, related to the hallucinations, and can influence behavior.

Memory loss is common, though relatively mild compared to Alzheimer's disease. However, periods of overt confusion and speech problems increase as the disease advances. Difficulty with executive function, planning, problem solving and initiating action may be more noticeable than in Alzheimer's. Visuo-spatial impairment is often prominent, with affected individuals getting lost, unable to do jigsaw puzzles or draw. Inattention and poor judgement are common symptoms as well, with patients usually lacking insight about their deficiencies. They are frequently indecisive and rigid in their thinking.

REM sleep behavior disorder is also present in many patients with DLB.[11] (REM is the rapid eye movement phase of sleep when we dream.) In this disturbing condition, patients appear to act out dream experiences, perhaps perceiving them as real. Sudden jerks or thrashing out of an extremity may occur, or more complex activity simulating walking, running or fighting, which may result in injury to the dreamer or his or her bed mate. REM sleep behavior disorder appears to be related to diseases where there is an accumulation of alpha-synuclein protein, which includes Parkinson's as well as dementia with Lewy bodies.

Whatever cognitive dysfunction is seen in DLB, the frequent presence of concomitant Alzheimer's must be kept in mind. Depression may also be a confounding element.

Observing the patient with DLB, the signs of Parkinsonism may be obvious, or so subtle as to almost be hidden during the early stages, and in some individuals, distinguishable only to the trained eye. Gait impairment is common. The patient may take small, shuffling steps and walk with a stooped or flexed posture, the body stiff and the normal arm swing decreased or absent. The individual may suddenly "freeze" while walking and be unable to move, seemingly glued to the ground. Rigidity of the extremities is noted when they are shifted passively, with abrupt releases and renewals known as "cogwheeling." There is difficulty with mobility and slowness of activity labeled as bradykinesia. Fine movements such as buttoning and handwriting may be also be impaired. Resting tremor, emblematic of Parkinson's disease, may be absent, or minimal when it does occur.

Myoclonic jerks, sudden twitches or jerks of an extremity or the whole body, are not uncommon in DLB. A significant percentage of these patients also have what is called autonomic dysfunction.[12] This indicates problems with the self-regulating systems in the body, such as blood pressure, bladder and bowel control, sexual function and sweating. Dizzy spells related to drops in blood pressure may result from this, along with incontinence and impotence.

TREATMENT

Aside from general measures, treatment targets three separate aspects of the disease (see Table 5.2).

General measures include the use of antioxidants such as vitamin E and possibly the monoamine oxidase-B inhibitor selegiline. There is no hard

Table 5.2
Treatment of DLB

1) Cognitive difficulties
2) Parkinsonian signs and symptoms
3) Behavioral problems

data confirming their efficacy. A baby aspirin and folic acid are probably also worthwhile to reduce the incidence of small strokes and improve circulation to the brain. Safety precautions are important because of the risk of falls and injuries, and the possibility of aspiration in the later stages.

The cholinesterase inhibitors used in Alzheimer's disease also have a role in DLB. These medications include Donepezil, rivastigmine and galantamine, and increase the availability of the neurotransmitter acetylcholine at the synaptic connections between neurons. Some of the stabilization or improvement in cognitive ability may be because of coexisting Alzheimer's in many patients, but these medications may work in pure DLB as well. However, if they do work, their effectiveness may be minor and temporary. There is not much data on treatment with memantine, but a trial of this drug may be considered.

The medications used for Parkinson's disease, dopa-agonists (drugs that act like levodopa) or levodopa itself in combination with enzymes that increase its availability in the brain, can be used to treat the motor abnormalities of DLB. Unfortunately, they are not as effective as in Parkinson's disease and may increase confusion and hallucinations. Because of this, it is necessary to achieve a balance when utilizing these drugs, giving enough so that the patients can walk and manage some of their daily tasks, while not causing too much confusion and disorientation. This is particularly important to assist caregivers and allow these patients to remain at home as long as possible.

Behavioral disturbances and agitation may also be difficult to treat. Some of the standard medications used for psychosis (neuroleptics) can worsen cognitive and motor function in patients with DLB, and so choosing the right drug is extremely important. The atypical antipsychotics such as risperidone, olanzapine or quetiapine are preferred, but their effectiveness varies. To help with sleep, clonazepam or desipramine may be employed. The question of whether to treat a patient's hallucinations depends on the individual case. If they are causing agitation or delusional behavior that may be dangerous, then treatment is certainly warranted.

If a patient is not bothered by his or her visions, and they are not threatening in any way, therapy may be held in abeyance.

Depression that interferes with functioning may warrant a trial of SSRI (selective serotonin uptake inhibitor) drugs, such as Zoloft, Celexa, Lexapro, etc. This should be monitored carefully to be sure there are no significant adverse effects.

Case History

Mike, an 80-year-old retired businessman, came for neurologic evaluation in May of 2003. He had seen a neurologist in another state six months earlier because of softness of his voice, slowness in walking and stooped posture which had started a year and a half earlier. His family also described problems with memory. CT scan had revealed atrophy and extensive blood work had been normal. There was a past history of prostate cancer for which he was receiving hormone injections. The neurologist noted fluctuating drowsiness along with dementia and Parkinsonian findings, and a diagnosis was made of Lewy body disease. He had been started on galantamine which the family felt had not helped. Subsequently, he and his wife had moved to an assisted living residence in Connecticut because their daughter was nearby.

When seen in May of 2003, he described shaking of his arms with activity, but not at rest. He had difficulty getting out of a chair, turning over in bed and problems dressing. Balance was impaired and he had periods of freezing where he could not move. Recent memory had become quite poor and he had gotten lost at times in his home. Occasional urinary incontinence was also occurring. He complained a lot about burning and tingling in the front of both thighs and his wife said that he slept a lot during the day. Of interest, his wife described vivid nightmares and sleep problems starting twenty years earlier which had continued.

On examination, the patient was disoriented to time, but knew the president and vice president. He could not perform simple calculations and could recall none of the three objects he was told to remember. His MMSE score was 18/30. Gait was slow with a flexed posture, decreased arm swing and tiny, shuffling steps. There was difficulty with fine movements and slight cogwheel rigidity. The patient also had an expressionless face and his speech was low in volume. Mild weakness of the hip flexor muscles were present with diminished vibration sense in his legs. The presumptive diagnosis was dementia with Lewy bodies and a possible neuropathy (damage to the nerves in his legs).

While we were waiting for his tests, he was started on L-dopa/carbidopa to treat the motor symptoms of his Parkinsonism and the galantamine 12 mg twice a day was continued. A baby aspirin was also added to his regimen. An MRI of the brain revealed generalized atrophy, perhaps more prominent frontally, and small vessel disease. EMGs confirmed the presence of a peripheral neuropathy and blood work was again normal. Because of concern about his cognitive status, his anti-Parkinsonian medications were raised very slowly.

By the end of June, Mike was taking L-dopa/carbidopa 25/100 three times a day. His memory and confusion had improved significantly according to the family. Walking and balance were also better, but he continued to sleep a lot during the day. On examination, he was fully oriented and could recall three of three objects at five and ten minutes. MMSE was 23. Medications were left unchanged. A month later, his walking was even better with cognitive ability the same. In November, it was noted that cognitive improvement had been maintained, though the family was aware of fluctuation and some periods of confusion. They also mentioned occasional jerks of his extremities while sleeping. There were no changes on examination.

When seen in January of 2004, his wife described increasing confusion and some visual hallucinations which did not bother him. Occasional myoclonic jerks occurred while sleeping, but walking and balance remained fairly good. On examination, some increase in flexed posture and reduction in arm swing were observed, and he did not know the year. But in March, he was improved from a cognitive standpoint, being fully oriented and with good short-term memory. His walking was slightly better. Fatigue and sleepiness remained a problem according to his wife. A mild stimulant, Provigil, was added to his medication, but his wife stopped it after two weeks because it was not helping. By May, his wife said he was hallucinating every day, seeing people outside the house and bugs on the floor. Though aware he was hallucinating, it did not make him anxious. Intermittent confusion and sleepiness persisted. On exam, he did not know the month or the president and could remember only one of three objects at five minutes. His motor findings were about the same.

In July, his wife stated he was more unsteady and slower in all activities. He complained of lightheadedness at times, and there were problems with fine movements and dressing. When questioned, he was not oriented to time, or exact place, and remembered one of three objects at five minutes. His gait was much slower, with no arm swing. It was quite difficult for him to get out of a chair and more cogwheeling was present.

Blood pressure was 95/60 sitting and 90/55 standing, with pulses of 86. His family was told to increase his salt and fluid intake, and L-dopa/carbidopa was raised to four times a day. In August, his walking and motor activity were improved, but the family said his confusion and hallucinations were worse. His blood pressure was in the same range on examination and he was fully oriented. The family was again told to increase his salt intake which they had not done.

At the end of September, his hallucinations had increased and some agitation was noted. His cognition continued to fluctuate: periods of confusion and forgetfulness alternating with intervals of relative clarity. In the office, his motor activity and walking were fairly good and blood pressure was 105/65 sitting and 95/65 standing. Because of the hallucinations and agitation, his L-dopa/carbidopa was reduced to three times daily. By early November, his confusion was worse, he was having some paranoid thoughts and hallucinations were more frequent. He was no longer able to dress himself and the lightheadedness remained. On examination, he was disoriented to time and place and could remember none of three objects. His gait was felt to be unchanged and blood pressures were the same as on the previous visit. After discussion with the family, his L-dopa/carbidopa was further reduced to twice daily and florinef was added to see if that would increase his blood pressure.

By mid-December, the family wanted to return to the higher dose of L-dopa/carbidopa. His walking was much worse and he had fallen several times. The confusion and hallucinations remained at the same level, but the family was having trouble caring for him because of his motor difficulties. In early January of 2005, the patient's legs began to swell and his shoes would not fit. The florinef was discontinued, as it was thought to be responsible.

L-dopa/carbidopa was increased to four times daily at the family's request in February, since they were having more problems managing him at the lower dose. Furosemide, a diuretic, had been started by his internist because of the swelling in his legs. When seen in April 2005, he was more confused, with some paranoid thoughts and almost continuous hallucinations. His walking seemed to be slightly better. By the end of June, the confusion and hallucinations were worse and he was sleeping much of the day. Some urinary incontinence had started and he had complained to his family of feeling as if he might black out. Exam was the same except that his blood pressure had dropped to 90/55 sitting and 80/50 standing. The diuretic was stopped and he was to return for a blood pressure check in a week.

He subsequently fell and broke his hip, and was placed in a nursing home.

PARKINSON'S DISEASE DEMENTIA

Most people associate Parkinson's disease with motor problems, particularly shaking of the hands and difficulty walking. Unfortunately, more than just the motor systems of the brain are involved, and cognitive impairment is common. This condition was first described by a general practitioner in London named James Parkinson in 1817,[13] and was known as paralysis agitans, or shaking palsy. A progressive degenerative disease, it ultimately led to immobilization and death until the 1970s, when L-dopa, the first effective treatment, began to be utilized. Since then, there have been a number of advances in therapy that slow the progression of the disease and allow patients to function, sometimes for many years. Eventually, however, there is less response to medications and patients become increasingly disabled.

While describing the gamut of symptoms and treatments employed in Parkinson's disease, we are going to focus particularly on the cognitive problems. It should be kept in mind, however, that when cognitive difficulties arise, the picture looks very similar to dementia with Lewy bodies and we may not duplicate all the information given in the preceding section.

DEMOGRAPHICS AND GENETICS

The prevalence of Parkinson's disease in the general population has been estimated to be about 384 cases per 100,000 people in North America.[14] For a population of 300 million in the United States, that would mean approximately 1,150,000 cases. Of course, in older age groups, the prevalence is much higher. In a European study, there were 1,800 cases of Parkinson's disease per 100,000 people 65 and older, and 2,600 cases per 100,000 from ages 85–89.[15] The lifetime risk of developing Parkinson's is estimated to be 4.4 percent for men and 3.7 percent for women, and it is believed there is a slight preponderance of the disease in men. About 5 percent of total cases occur in persons under 40. Of interest, mild Parkinsonian signs, but not Parkinson's disease, have been found in up to 40 percent of older people living in the community.[16]

It has been suggested that certain personality types have a higher likelihood of developing Parkinson's: those individuals who are highly organized, parsimonious, phlegmatic, introspective and cautious. Anxiety and pessimism early in life may also be associated with a higher risk of Parkinson's disease later on.[17] But rather than increasing the chances of developing Parkinson's, it is possible that some common factor underlies these traits and the disease itself. Depression is also seen frequently in

Parkinson's patients before the onset of motor symptoms, but the relationship between the two conditions is unclear. Certainly after the disease becomes manifest, depression would not be unexpected. Estimates of the presence of dementia in patients with Parkinson's disease are generally in the range of 30–50 percent, though they have been as high as 70 percent.

Twenty years ago, some investigators in the field supported the idea that exposure to unknown environmental toxins caused Parkinson's. This was not borne out and a genetic origin for the disease subsequently became popular. However, this hypothesis was also not substantiated, even though familial forms of the disease are well known. The likelihood is that a combination of genetic predisposition and environmental factors are responsible for this disorder. The chances of having Parkinson's at age 80 is about 2 percent in the general population and 5–6 percent if a parent or sibling was affected.[18] When both a parent and sibling have had the disease, the chances of developing it increase to between 20 and 40 percent.

A number of families have been found where specific genetic abnormalities cause Parkinson's disease. But for the vast majority of people with this illness, so-called idiopathic Parkinson's, no firm hereditary basis has been established. In one important grouping of patients, a mutation in the gene for alpha-synuclein, the main component of Lewy bodies, was found to result in Parkinson's, inherited in an autosomal dominant fashion. Most investigators feel alpha-synuclein plays a critical role in the story of Parkinsons's disease, but it is not clear exactly what that is. The aggregation or clumping of alpha-synuclein may be considered as being similar to that of beta-amyloid in Alzheimer's disease, and may be responsible for synapatic disruption, neuronal dysfunction and eventually cell death. Cases have also been discovered inherited as autosomal recessives involving the parkin gene, as well as ubiquitin genes. Most of the early onset cases appear to have genetic links, though some may also be drug induced, caused by compounds such as MPTP. A great deal of work is currently under way to try and paint the entire genetic picture of Parkinson's, with the hope this will lead to more effective treatments in the future.

PATHOLOGICAL FEATURES

The brain of a person with Parkinson's disease at autopsy may appear normal, or show mild atrophy of the frontal lobes. However, when the brain is sectioned, one sees a characteristic finding—the loss of pigmented neurons in a deep part of the brain called the substantia nigra. (The substantia nigra is a dark stripe on both sides of the base of the brain whose cells contain neuromelanin pigment as well as the neurotransmitter dopamine.) The cells here send impulses to higher centers in the brain involved with motor activity and when dysfunctional or dying can cause problems with walking, balance, muscle tone and tremor.

The other hallmark of Parkinson's is the presence of Lewy bodies that have previously been described. In Parkinson's disease, their distribution is different than in DLB, with a preponderance in the brain stem and deep structures, rather than the cerebral cortex. However, they are present in the cortex in increasing amounts as the disease progresses, particularly when dementia occurs. In fact, there is a correlation between widespread Lewy bodies in the cortex, particularly the medial temporal lobe, and the presence of dementia.[19] The pathologic changes of Alzheimer's disease may also coexist in Parkinsonian patients, senile plaques more than neurofibrillary tangles, and may be partially responsible for the dementia when it is seen. But the cognitive impairment also happens independently, probably related to the presence of the Lewy bodies. Though a decrease in the neurotransmitter dopamine is the biochemical change responsible for the motor dysfunction in Parkinson's, there are also lower amounts of the neurotransmitter acetylcholine, and this may be an important factor in the development of dementia. This "cholinergic deficit" may explain the response of Parkinson's dementia patients to cholinesterase inhibitors that increase the amount of acetylcholine available at the synapses in the brain.

DIAGNOSTIC EVALUATION AND CLINICAL PICTURE

Parkinson's disease is basically a clinical diagnosis, meaning that in most cases a physician can make the diagnosis by history, observation and examination, without additional studies (see Table 5.3). However, certain tests may be helpful in excluding conditions similar to Parkinson's, or

Table 5.3
Diagnostic Features of Parkinson's Disease

1) Tremor
2) Rigidity
3) Bradykinesia
4) Postural instability

Source: Douglas Gelb et al., "Diagnostic Criteria for Parkinson's Disease," *Arch Neurol,* 1999, 54: 33–39.

present concurrently. Autopsy studies of patients who were diagnosed clinically as having Parkinson's only confirmed the diagnosis in about 65 to 80 percent of cases,[20] though specialists in movement disorders were correct 98.6 percent of the time. Thus, as expected, the expertise of the examiner determines the accuracy of the diagnosis.

The abnormalities noted in Table 5.3 are emblematic of Parkinson's disease[21] and when all are seen the diagnosis is usually straight forward. Yet even when all or most of these findings are present, up to one-quarter may have another condition responsible.

The tremor of Parkinson's disease is seen in the lower portion of one or both arms, but can also involve the legs. Typically it is present at rest and has been noted in 79 to 90 percent of patients with the disease.[22] However, it can occur in other illnesses that mimic Parkinson's.

Rigidity (increased muscle tone and stiffness) is found in 89 to 99 percent of Parkinson's patients, but also in a number of similar disorders.

Bradykinesia is a slowness of movement. Though it has been reported in 77 to 98 percent of individuals with Parkinson's, it can occur in a multiplicity of other conditions, including normal aging, depression and Alzheimer's, as well as Parkinson's-like diseases.

Postural instability (difficulty maintaining upright position) tends to develop later in the course of the disease.

Asymmetrical onset of symptoms is expected in Parkinson's, though occasionally both sides can be involved early.

Problems with speech are almost universal, with low volume, inability to project and occasional slurring. Difficulty swallowing is a frequent symptom as the disease progresses.

Depression can be seen in up to 40 percent of cases, though severe in only 8 percent.

When patients are treated with L-dopa or similar drugs, as many as 20 percent may experience hallucinations, generally when the disease is more advanced.

Autonomic problems, as described in DLB, are not uncommon in Parkinson's. These include drop in blood pressure with dizziness when standing, constipation, urinary urgency and frequency, sweating and sexual dysfunction.

Freezing is also found in many Parkinsonian patients, where the feet are fixed to the ground and the person is unable to move.

MRI and CT scans are usually not helpful in diagnosis, because there is no specific pattern seen on these studies. However, they can assist in excluding other conditions that might confuse the picture, such as strokes or tumors in particular areas of the brain. In Parkinson's patients with dementia, atrophy of the medial temporal lobe was found to be even more pronounced than in Alzheimer's on MRI,[23] but this is of no value in making a diagnosis.

SPECT scans and PET scans may be of assistance in diagnosing Parkinson's disease in those patients whose clinical presentation is unclear, though their main application so far has been in experimental studies. PET and SPECT scans using specific radioactive markers have unique patterns in Parkinson's disease, with diminished uptake of these chemicals (and less radioactivity on the scans) in a deep part of the brain called the striatum, or basal ganglia.[24] These markers are concentrated in neurons that produce the neurotransmitter dopamine, and as those cells become impaired or die off, less of the chemicals are bound at these sites. Thus there is an inverse relationship between the degree of motor dysfunction in Parkinson's disease and the presence of these chemicals in the basal ganglia.

There are no blood tests that aid in the diagnosis, and spinal taps are not helpful.

As mentioned previously, dementia affects anywhere from 30 to 70 percent of individuals with Parkinson's, depending on how carefully cognitive evaluations are performed and how long the patients are followed. One study found that 26 percent of Parkinson's patients had some evidence of dementia when they were first seen.[25] Within 4 years, this had increased to 51 percent and at 8 years, the prevalence of dementia was nearly 80 percent. (However, we must also keep in mind that if dementia is present early on with motor symptoms, it may be due to DLB rather than Parkinson's.) Age in an important risk factor for Parkinson's patients developing dementia: the older they are, the more likely they are to become demented. Other risk factors include duration and severity of the disease and the presence of postural problems, gait abnormalities and medication induced hallucinations.[26] Severe head trauma can probably be added to the list as well. And many Parkinsonian patients who are not demented are likely to have some degree of cognitive impairment.[27]

The dementia of Parkinson's disease has been labeled a "subcortical dementia" because the deep structures of the brain are involved earlier and disproportionately to the cerebral cortex as seen in Alzheimer's and fronto-temporal dementia. However, it may be difficult to differentiate the two types clinically, and by the time dementia occurs in Parkinson's, there is usually considerable involvement of cortical neurons. So the term "subcortical dementia" may be at least partially a misnomer. Pathological studies have shown a loss of neurons consistently in deep brain structures in Parkinson's patients with dementia, along with diminished stores of a chemical important in the production of acetylcholine (choline acetyltransferase) in regions of the cerebral cortex.[28] The latter deficit is similar to that seen in Alzheimer's, though the typical plaques and tangles may not always be present.

The same pattern of cognitive impairment seen in dementia with Lewy bodies also occurs in Parkinson's disease dementia, though hallucinations may be less frequent. Often, when hallucinations develop, they are associated with levodopa use, or a dopa agonist, or an increase in dosage, and may disappear when the medication is stopped or reduced. Difficulties with memory and executive function are prominent. It has been said that patients with Parkinson's dementia have particular problems with retrieval and recall, but good recognition, and that these problems are present with both recent and remote memory.[29] This differs from Alzheimer's where patients do not store information and thus cannot recall it later, even if they are given clues. Speech impairment is often a major feature, but usually because of motor dysfunction rather than language derangement. Visuo-spatial problems are also found frequently and are more severe than in Alzheimer's.[30]

As in DLB, fluctuation of cognitive symptoms and attention also occurs in Parkinson's dementia. Neuropsychiatric symptoms are common, as is REM sleep behavior disorder. Depression is more frequent in patients with Parkinson's dementia than in Parkinson's alone, and agitation, delusions and behavioral disturbances may all be part of the picture. Again, medications may bring these symptoms to the fore, or exacerbate them when they have been present previously.

TREATMENT

For the past 40 years, the standard treatment for Parkinson's disease has been levodopa. This is still the most important therapeutic agent, but its use has been enhanced in a number of ways. It is generally given now in combination with an another compound (carbidopa) that prevents its breakdown outside the nervous system and increases its availability to the cells in the brain that use dopamine as a neurotransmitter— levodopa/carbidopa pills. Another advance has been to administer the medications in a controlled release pill that delivers a steady stream of levodopa to the neurons, eliminating any pulsatile (up and down) effects that may have adverse consequences. In the past few years, other compounds have been employed to further increase levodopa's availability to the neurons and extend its effectiveness (COMT inhibitors-catechol-O-methyltransferase).

Another class of medications helpful in treating Parkinson's has been the dopa-agonists (Mirapex-pramipexole, Requip-ropinirole). These medications act like levodopa in the brain and are often useful in the early stages of the disease. Some investigators believe that responsiveness to levodopa lasts for a limited amount of time and by employing dopa-agonists as long as possible at the beginning, the benefits of levodopa later on can be extended. They also feel dopa-agonists may provide neuroprotection to the neurons that produce dopamine. This would be particularly worthwhile in younger patients who will have to take these medications for many years. However, these concepts are only theoretical and when patients begin to have motor problems that interfere with their quality of life, levodopa is more effective than dopa-agonists. The latter medications can also be utilized in combination with levodopa and may reduce the amount of "off-time" when patients have difficulty with motor activity.

Amantadine (Symmetrel) has been used in Parkinson's for about 30 years. It was originally employed as an antiviral agent to prevent influenza until observers realized it also seemed to improve Parkinsonian patients. Amantadine is one of the minor or supplementary drugs and appears to be helpful in reducing tremor. At times, it may also decrease the abnormal movements (dyskinesias, chorea) that can result from levodopa or dopa-agonist therapy.

Selegiline (Eldepryl, Deprenyl) is one of a class of drugs called selective MAO-B inhibitors. Believed to have neuroprotective effects, it combats oxidative stress and free radicals and shields cells from neurotoxic damage caused by certain chemicals. (It has been used as well in Alzheimer's for neuroprotection.) Selegiline may also work to a minimal degree in lessening Parkinsonian symptoms. Overall, it appears to have minor benefits, though some similar compounds are now being tested. One of these, rasagiline may be helpful in reducing "off" time and freezing in moderately advanced Parkinson's patients.

Coenzyme Q10, which protects mitochondrial function within the cells and is a strong antioxidant, has been used experimentally in the treatment of early Parkinson's disease and appeared to slow progressive functional decline.[31] Further studies are necessary to define its efficacy and how it should be employed.

Though anticholinergic drugs have been utilized to treat Parkinson's disease for about 100 years, they have fallen by the wayside for the most part as new and more effective drugs have become available. They also have numerous side effects that limit their usefulness in older patients and those with cognitive compromise.

Surgical therapy now has to be considered in individuals with very severe motor symptoms inadequately controlled by medications. In the past, certain deep bodies of nerve cells within the brain (globus pallidus or thalamus) were destroyed to reduce tremor. Currently, deep brain stimulators are being implanted to modify activity of these cells without destroying them. The results of these procedures are variable.

The placement of stem cells into the brain of Parkinson's patients to replace neurons that were damaged or destroyed is an avenue that offers promise for future therapy. At present, however, the technique is not advanced enough to provide immediate benefits in patients who are severely deteriorated.

When treating Parkinsonian patients with dementia, the cholinesterase inhibitors given in Alzheimer's and DLB may provide some modest benefits (Donepezil-Aricept, rivastigmine-Exelon, galantamine-Reminyl) as shown in a recent large study with rivastigmine.[32] Patients were able to function better, with improvement or less decline in the activities of daily living, than control groups. Neuropsychiatric symptoms improved and some patients also had temporary increases in MMSE scores. However, gastrointestinal side effects and worsening of motor symptoms were seen as well. These medications act by preventing the breakdown of acetylcholine and increasing its availability as a neurotransmitter at the synapses.

The value of memantine (Namenda) in Parkinson's dementia is unknown, but may be worth trying if there are significant cognitive problems.

The use of medications to treat psychiatric and behavioral symptoms requires caution, as standard antipsychotic agents, as in DLB, may produce worsening of Parkinson's. The atypical antipsychotic drugs risperidone, olanzapine or quetiapine may provide the best results. Clonazepam or desipramine may be used when there are problems with sleep. Depression can be treated with SSRIs (selective serotonin uptake inhibitors) such as Zoloft, Celexa, Lexapro, etc, with the patient watched for any adverse effects.

When treating Parkinson's patients with dementia, neuropsychiatric or behavioral problems, one of the considerations must always be a reduction of levodopa, dopa-agonists and other anti-Parkinsonian medications, as these can cause cognitive and psychiatric symptoms or make them worse when they are present. As with DLB, use of these medications often requires balancing a patient's motor abilities against cognitive dysfunction, with the families helping to decide what is necessary to allow them to continue care.

While offering some symptomatic relief, with possible temporary stabilization of cognitive decline, the cholinesterase inhibitors and other current medications do not affect the basic disease process or progression of the dementia. Better understanding of the role of alpha synuclein and Lewy bodies in Parkinson's disease dementia and DLB will be necessary before more effective strategies can be devised to halt or reverse these diseases.

Case History

James was a 78-year-old man seen for neurologic evaluation in May of 1997. His major complaint was shaking of his right hand, present for nine months, mainly at rest. He also had rare shaking of his jaw and minor difficulty with handwriting. Being an artist, he had difficulty working because of some incoordination. Walking and balance were uncompromised and there was no significant medical history. Examination revealed a slight decrease of right arm swing while walking, mild tremulousness of both arms and a moderate resting tremor of the right arm. There was also some cogwheel rigidity of the right wrist and slight facial masking. The diagnosis was early Parkinson's disease and the patient was started on Amantadine for the tremor and a baby aspirin. An MRI showed small vessel disease.

The tremor was reduced on this regimen and the patient was satisfied. In January of 1998, Selegiline 5 mg twice a day and Vitamin E 1,000 IU daily were added. Examination in April showed no tremor, but slight facial masking and right wrist cogwheel rigidity. He said that when he was nervous, the shaking returned. Throughout the remainder of 1998 and 1999, the patient did well, with intermittent tremor of the right arm. In February of 2000, he noted some difficulty with balance and said that he had stopped playing golf. There were also minor problems getting out of a chair and turning over in bed. However, he felt he was not limited and did not want additional medications. Examination showed a Parkinsonian tremor of the right arm with some increased rigidity in both arms, but was otherwise unchanged.

By September, James was noted to have a flexed posture and a slight shuffling gait in addition to his other findings, but insisted on the same regimen. He continued to progress slowly through April of 2001, when he was found to have difficulty turning and more problems with balance. His handwriting had also deteriorated. At this point, he agreed to try prami-pexole and was begun on 0.25 mg three time daily. Selegiline was stopped. However, the patient became extremely sleepy on pramipexole, dropping off at inopportune times. Some mild confusion was also described by his wife and the pramipexole was discontinued. On the next examination at the end of May, the patient's motor findings were unchanged and he appeared cognitively intact, with an MMSE of 29. An avid bridge player, he was having no problems remembering the cards and played regularly. He was now started on levodopa/carbidopa CR 50/200 twice a day. A week later, his wife called to say that he was having a lot of bad dreams, moving his legs and flailing his arms at night. But he was better during the day in terms of his motor symptoms. Clonazepam 0.25 mg at bedtime was added.

When seen in July, James admitted to minor problems with memory and feeling slightly off balance. He was also stammering, but said that his shaking and fine movements were better. His nightmares had stopped. Examination did confirm a slight improvement and his medications were continued, apart from Amantadine which was decreased to twice a day. Over the next several months he remained stable, both from a motor and cognitive standpoint and was able to function fairly well.

In March of 2002, the patient and his wife noted that he was able to paint again, which he had stopped a number of months earlier. There were no cognitive problems and his bridge game was fine. Examination was basically unchanged. When seen in July, he said he had only been taking his levodopa/carbidopa once a day instead of twice because he felt that was all he needed. On exam, however, his walking was worse and he had trouble arising from a chair. His right-sided tremor was more pronounced and his speech much softer. He was strongly advised to take his medication twice a day. By October however, he had progressed further. Though unchanged cognitively, he was walking more stiffly, with a flexed posture and decreased arm swing, and had difficulty getting out of a chair. His tremor, cogwheel rigidity and fine movements had all worsened, as had his speech and handwriting. The dosage of levodopa/carbidopa was increased to three times daily.

At the end of November, all motor activity was improved and there was no change in cognition. Medication was left the same and the patient remained stable through August of 2003. In September, his wife called to say he was talking a lot in his sleep, was restless and was keeping her up. There was no confusion or significant problems with memory.

She asked if she could raise his dose of clonazepam to 0.5 mg at night and was told she could, but was told to watch for any cognitive changes. The increase in clonazepam seemed to help his sleeping and he had no adverse effects. Through the rest of 2003 and early 2004, he did well in terms of his Parkinson's disease, but developed pain in his calves while walking due to peripheral vascular disease, confirmed by Doppler ultrasound. His primary care physician did not suggest medication or intervention and the patient was content to live with his discomfort. He continued to play bridge regularly.

By May of 2004, there was increased difficulty arising from a chair and turning over in bed. His balance was off and he had fallen several times. On rare occasions, he froze while walking. Cognitive problems were denied and his score on the MMSE was 25. His levodopa/carbidopa was raised to four times a day. In July of 2004, his motor abilities had improved slightly, but he was having more nightmares and occasional periods of confusion. His clonazepam was reduced to 0.25 mg at bedtime. Through December, he remained fairly stable, with less nightmares and periods of confusion. His MMSE in December was 25.

In the early part of 2005, he continued to have intermittent confusion, his thought processes were slower and he had stopped playing bridge. There were no hallucinations. By mid-March, his wife noted increased freezing and worsening of motor activity, and she was having more difficulty caring for him, even with a part-time aide. On examination, he was very stiff and moved slowly, shuffling and taking small steps. His tremor and rigidity seemed the same. He was fully oriented but could remember only one of three objects and his MMSE was 24. The levodopa/carbidopa was increased to five times a day with the warning that his cognitive problems might escalate. But by mid-April, he seemed slightly better and was getting physical therapy.

Over the next month, he deteriorated further. Lexapro 5 mg daily (an antidepressant) was added by his internist. He was using a walker in the house and a wheelchair for transportation outside. He was freezing when he tried to walk and almost fell on numerous occasions. His shaking was worse and he could neither turn over in bed unaided nor get up from a chair. There were problems with fine movements and his handwriting was barely legible. Intermittent confusion and problems with memory continued, but no hallucinations. Mild dyskinesia (abnormal twisting movements) was observed for the first time. He was fully oriented, knew the president and vice-president, and could remember two of three objects after five minutes. It was decided to add ropinerole (a dopa-agonist)

0.25 mg four times daily to his medications to see if that would help his motor symptoms.

His wife called a week later to say that he was much more confused and agitated. He had never started the ropinerole because it had been too much trouble with his other medications. The levodopa/carbidopa was reduced to three times daily and his Amantadine lowered to once each morning. Three weeks later his wife said his agitation was gone and he was less confused. However, he could not walk because of poor balance and frequent freezing. His shaking and other symptoms remained the same. Examination revealed difficulty following commands and recall of only one of three objects. But he was fully oriented and knew the president and vice-president. Walking was very unsteady with severe impairment of postural mechanisms and a tendency to fall backward or off to the side if he were not caught. There was minimal dyskinesia. To try and improve his walking, his levodopa/carbidopa was increased to four times daily and his wife told to call in two weeks.

Chapter 6

VASCULAR DEMENTIA AND MIXED DEMENTIA

The slips that my memory has so often made, even when it was most confident of itself, have not been wasted on me. In vain does it swear to me and assure me now; I just shake my head . . . and I should not dare to rely on it for anything of importance.

Montaigne[1]

Looking back at the beach
even my footprints are gone.

Ozaki Hosai[2]

Most older people have some vascular changes in the brain, though the degree of involvement varies. When dementia from any cause occurs in the elderly, it is likely that cerebrovascular disease is playing some role and a more accurate label for many of these cases might be mixed dementia.[3] Similarly, when vascular disease bears major responsibility for cognitive deterioration, Alzheimer's plaques and tangles or Lewy bodies can usually be found as well. Though Lewy bodies and other pathology are seen together with vascular changes, the term mixed dementia is currently used for Alzheimer's and vascular disease coexisting in the brain. This chapter will focus on those patients whose cerebrovascular disease is the main driver of dementia, as well as those who have a mixed picture. Vascular dementia has also been called multi-infarct dementia and post-stroke dementia.

When we speak of cerebrovascular disease, we mean atherosclerotic changes in the arteries that supply the brain, depriving brain tissue of blood (ischemia), or causing death of brain tissue (infarction). Atherosclerosis is a build-up of fatty materials in the arteries that reduces blood flow through narrowing (stenosis) or obstruction (complete blockage).

DEMOGRAPHICS, GENETICS AND RISK FACTORS

Dealing with two such common conditions, cerebrovascular disease and dementia, it is hard to give accurate statistics about their interrelationship, and how often vascular disease "causes" cognitive dysfunction, because as noted, different processes may be affecting the brain simultaneously. In addition, tracking cerebrovascular disease can present problems because of the various forms it takes; from massive strokes that suddenly generate severe brain damage and neurological impairment, to tiny silent strokes that may go unrecognized; involving major blood vessels supplying large areas of the brain, to small arteries and arterioles responsible for minuscule portions of brain tissue. And when vascular injuries to the brain occur, they may be abrupt and produce irreversible deficits; or they may cause transient dysfunction that appears to return to normal but leaves minor alterations that may not be appreciated; or they may be silent until a particular threshold is reached and they become manifest clinically. As one report on the two conditions noted, "The diagnosis of vascular dementia is difficult in epidemiologic studies because poststroke dementia can be due to Alzheimer's disease and evidence of vascular disease can be found in the MRI of dementia cases without clinical strokes. Whether the clinical progression is related to Alzheimer's pathology or vascular disease is difficult to establish."[4]

Cerebrovascular disease may be the primary cause of dementia in 10–20 percent of cases and a major contributing factor in another 30–50 percent. In a study that evaluated over 3,300 older patients who were not demented and had MRIs, 13.3 percent developed dementia over the following six years. Of these, 44 percent were felt to be of possible or probable vascular origin.[5] Up to two-thirds of the patients who have had a stroke have some degree of cognitive impairment afterward, though not necessarily full dementia. But 25 percent of individuals who have dementia, have had previous strokes, a large percentage of which may be silent and discovered on imaging studies. There has been a suggestion that 20 percent of individuals over 60 have had at least one silent stroke. The incidence of cognitive impairment as well as dementia after a stroke increases as age increases.[6] The finding of white matter changes due to small vessel disease on MRI significantly increases the risk of developing dementia. Around 25–45 percent of patients with Alzheimer's have been shown to have considerable cerebrovascular disease pathologically.

Vascular dementia is probably the second most common cause of dementia in the United States, but the most common cause in Japan and other parts of Asia, the Soviet Union and Finland. The higher prevalence in these regions is undoubtably due to the higher rates of hypertension and stroke.

There is no particular genetic pattern associated with vascular dementia. However, any genetic predisposition to atherosclerosis, such as diabetes or hypertension, also increases the odds of developing a dementia of vascular origin.

The occurrence of vascular risk factors in midlife may actually be of greater consequence in terms of producing dementia in the future, than the presence of these elements later in life, though they are important there as well. This somewhat paradoxical effect may have to do with the cumulative changes they induce in the blood vessels over time, as well as the accrual of small and larger vascular lesions in the brain.

Analyzing the risk factors for vascular dementia listed in Table 6.1, we see they are the same as for Alzheimer's disease, or dementia in general. They also raise the chances of a future stroke or heart attack. In other words, we are speaking of all the determinants linked to atherosclerosis, for this is the basis of vascular dementia. Studies have shown that those risk factors predisposing to stroke are also associated with a greater likelihood of cognitive decline in older people.[7] In addition, excessive alcohol

Table 6.1
Risk Factors for Vascular Dementia

1) Hypertension
2) Diabetes
3) Elevated Cholesterol
4) Obesity
5) Sedentary Life Style
6) Previous Stroke
7) Previous Heart Attack
8) Presence of White Matter Lesions on MRI (small vessel disease)
9) Smoking
10) Atrial fibrillation (irregular heart rhythm)

intake increases the risk of vascular dementia as does the presence of the APOE 4 gene and elevated homocysteine levels in the blood.

It has also been proposed that comorbid medical conditions (other medical problems present at the same time) are an independent risk factor increasing the possibility of dementia after a stroke.[8] These other disorders, such as seizures, cardiac arrythmias and pneumonia, can reduce oxygen supply to the brain, compounding any damage caused by a stroke. Stroke survivors with these comorbid conditions had a much higher incidence of dementia than those without, almost 50 percent versus 22 percent after four and a half years of observation. Interestingly, another study showed that people with peripheral vascular disease (atherosclerosis involving the legs) had more cognitive deficits on neuropsychological testing than control subjects.[9] Their dysfunction was similar to that seen in patients with cerebrovascular disease, even though they had no clinical evidence of vascular problems involving the brain. It was assumed in this study that atherosclerosis in one area of the body was indicative of a more generalized process, and included diminished circulation to the brain causing cognitive compromise.

PATHOLOGY AND DIAGNOSTIC EVALUATION

Pathology

When examining the brains of patients with vascular dementia, some degree of atrophy is usually present along with evidence of focal damage caused by strokes (cerebral infarctions). The number and size of these lesions vary considerably from case to case. A few small strokes in critical areas may be enough to cause significant dementia in some patients, while others may be seen with multiple major strokes throughout the brain. Cerebral infarctions may be the result of large blood vessel occlusions, small blood vessel disease, clots that come from the heart (emboli) or a combination of these. In some cases, there may be a predominance of strokes in the cerebral cortex, while in other cases, they may be mainly in the deeper areas of the brain. The strokes may result in softening of the brain (encephalomalacia) or scarring. Looking at the brain tissue microscopically, there is confirmation of ischemic and hypoxic damage (diminished blood flow and oxygen). The cerebral arteries and arterioles (small arteries) show changes due to atherosclerosis and high blood pressure, with calcium deposits in the vessel walls, cholesterol and lipid plaques that obstruct the vessels and reduce blood flow, along with inflammation in the blood vessel walls. Clots may or may not be found in some of the arteries, but the platelets in the blood are noted to be more sticky and adherent, and the blood clots more easily.

A type of vascular dementia involving the white matter around the ventricles with multiple small areas of ischemia has been called Binswanger's disease after the physician who described it over a century ago, but its prevalence and clinical manifestations are still somewhat controversial.[10]

As mentioned, the incidence of concomitant pathology in the brain, such as Alzheimer's disease, or DLB, is high in patients with vascular dementia.

Diagnosis

The diagnosis of vascular dementia is made through a combination of history, examination and laboratory data. The history is usually of multiple strokes having occurred, with progressive deterioration of cognitive function accelerated by each event. Physical examination reveals cognitive compromise, but shows evidence of past strokes as well. This may include language problems (aphasia), motor or sensory deficits, visual impairment or difficulty with walking and balance.

Imaging studies, such as an MRI or CT scan, are of prime importance in establishing the diagnosis, for the presence of strokes must be confirmed. The number, size and location of the strokes are different in each case, but they are always multiple and can be visualized. Invariably, one finds the ubiquitous changes of small vessel ischemic disease in the white matter of the brain as well. SPECT or PET scans can also be used to demonstrate the deficits. Vascular studies that look directly at the blood vessels are not necessary to make a diagnosis, but may be of value in deciding on treatment. These tests include carotid doppler (ultrasound) studies to look at the carotid arteries, MRA (magnetic resonance angiography) and CT angiography.

Excluding cardiac causes for strokes may also be important, as clots can travel from the heart to the brain as emboli, block the blood vessels and cause damage. An echocardiogram and other tests may provide the required information. And once a diagnosis of vascular dementia has been made, the presence of vascular risk factors should be sought, which means tests for diabetes and lipid profile, homocysteine levels, C-reactive protein and sedimentation rate.

CLINICAL PICTURE

The typical age of onset for vascular dementia is between 60 and 75, with a slight predominance in men. Along with the variability in size, number and location of the strokes, the clinical picture in each case varies as well. The classic description is of a stepwise deterioration in cognitive function, heralding the occurrence of new strokes. The patient has an episode followed by cognitive decline, then stabilizes for awhile. Then there is a new stroke and intellectual function is a bit worse. The patient plateaus again for awhile longer and then another event occurs. And this pattern continues until the patient is severely demented, with or without accompanying neurologic deficits.

However, this expected picture is not always present. Not infrequently, there is a slow, progressive decline in cognitive ability similar to Alzheimer's disease, rather than a stepwise drop-off. The strokes may be silent, without sudden changes as the patient deteriorates. At times, one major or even minor stroke may be seen, followed by a progressive inexorable loss of intellectual function. Or a patient may slowly dwindle and then rapidly accelerate when another stroke occurs.

The parameters of cognitive dysfunction in vascular dementia depend on the location and severity of the previous strokes. A so-called subcortical dementia due to deep strokes may look different than one caused by strokes mainly involving the cerebral cortex. In addition, strokes predominantly in the right or left cerebral hemisphere produce diverse findings, as do those involving the language areas versus the regions for visuo-spatial functions. Thus, there is no predictable pattern for vascular dementia in terms of specific symptoms that are prevalent, or a particular time course.

Not withstanding the variability, the cognitive deficits in vascular dementia are similar to those described for other dementias. Memory is generally affected along with attention, executive function and language ability. Loss of visuo-spatial proficiency may occur as well and a fluctuating state with periods of confusion is not uncommon. When there is significant frontal lobe involvement, disinhibition and loss of social restraints may be seen. A global deterioration of all cognitive functions is another presentation.

Since all of these abnormalities can be found in Alzheimer's patients and the pathological processes may overlap, how do we differentiate between the two conditions? Though it may be difficult, there are certain features that point more toward a vascular origin for the dementia. A stepwise progression is one of them. The presence of strokes on imaging studies is another. A history of strokes or focal neurologic deficits on examination is also suggestive evidence. Motor weakness, problems walking, sensory deficits, visual field cuts, slurred speech, disproportionate problems with language all favor cerebrovascular disease if present early. Another unusual finding associated with strokes is "emotional incontinence": inappropriate crying or laughing by a patient that cannot be controlled, and is not in response to an expected stimulus.

There are established criteria set forth by different investigators in this field that have been used to confirm the diagnosis of vascular dementia versus other possible causes in someone with cognitive loss. One of these is the Hachinski ischemic score named for the originator as shown in Table 6.2.[11] A score of seven or more in a patient with dementia favors a vascular origin, while a score of four or less makes vascular dementia highly unlikely.

The clinical picture of mixed dementia can also be quite varied. The signs and symptoms are similar to those seen in vascular dementia, but with Alzheimer's tipping the scale. In addition to the number, location and severity of the strokes that help determine the presentation, there is the relative role of the Alzheimer's process coexisting in the brain to be taken into account. Whether Alzheimer's and vascular disease contribute equally to the dementia, or is it 90 percent Alzheimer's and 10 percent vascular, or vice versa, or any percentages in between, can make a difference in how the dementia presents and progresses, and in any associated findings.

Table 6.2
The Hachinski Ischemic Score

Item	Score value
Abrupt onset	2
Stepwise progression	1
Fluctuating course	2
Nocturnal confusion	1
Relative preservation of personality	1
Depression	1
Somatic complaints	1
Emotional incontinence	1
History of hypertension	1
History of strokes	2
Evidence of associated atherosclerosis	1
Focal neurological symptoms	2
Focal neurological signs	2

TREATMENT

There are two aspects of treating vascular dementia to be considered. One is combating the underlying processes of atherosclerosis and hypertension to try and prevent further vascular compromise and brain damage. The second is the treatment of the dementia itself to see if cognitive function and quality of life can be improved.

The standard steps to combat all types of vascular disease are also applicable for vascular dementia. If the individual is smoking, it should be stopped immediately. Blood pressure should be vigorously controlled with whatever intervention is required. Elevated cholesterol and triglycerides should be brought down into a normal range using diet, statin drugs and any other medications that might be helpful. If the affected person is capable of an exercise program, it should be started. He or she should be taking aspirin, or other medications that reduce platelet adhesiveness and clotting to lessen the possibility of recurrent strokes. If diabetes is present, that should also be tackled aggressively. Unfortunately, even if all of these factors are managed well, the dementing process once initiated may continue, with or without additional strokes.

Treating the dementia to try and improve memory and other cognitive functions, or at least halt the rapidity of decline, entails the use of cholinesterase inhibitors employed in Alzheimer's disease. Indeed, some neuroscientists believe that any positive effects from these compounds in vascular dementia is because the treatment is actually affecting the coexisting Alzheimer's process present in so many of these patients. However it works, patients with vascular dementia do appear to benefit from the use of these medications,[12] which increases the amount of the neurotransmitter acetylcholine available at certain synapses in the brain, slowing the rate of cognitive decline. As yet, there is no good data about the use of memantine in vascular dementia, but a trial of this in patients who are deteriorating would appear to be reasonable.

Prevention should be the main thrust in addressing vascular dementia, because once brain tissue is destroyed it cannot be regenerated or function restored. That means paying attention to vascular risk factors that may be present early in life and doing whatever is possible to eliminate them.

Case History

George was a 60-year-old man seen initially by another neurologist in the hospital in October of 2000 with a transient aphasia (problems speaking). He was supposed to have been on a blood thinner (coumadin) to protect against clots from the heart (emboli) because of an irregular heart beat (atrial fibrillation) but had been taking the medication erratically. There was also a history of coronary artery disease (atherosclerosis of the blood vessels of the heart). Examination revealed loss of vision in the right visual field, right facial weakness and slight difficulty with coordination in the right hand. Blood pressure was 130/80, pulse 74 and irregular. CT scan in the hospital showed a stroke on the left side of the brain involving the temporal and parietal lobes. His pro-time (a measure of efficacy of his blood thinner) confirmed that his coumadin level was low. Carotid doppler (ultrasound of the arteries) was normal. Within 48 hours, the patient's neurological abnormalities cleared and he was cognitively intact. His coumadin was restarted and he was discharged from the hospital, with an echocardiogram (ultrasound of the heart) to be scheduled as an outpatient.

Two weeks later, he was readmitted to the hospital with a seizure and left sided weakness. His pro-time was again below the therapeutic range and MRI of the brain showed multiple areas of infarction (strokes) in both hemispheres. There was also scattered small vessel disease that had not been appreciated on the previous CT scan. EEG monitoring showed an epileptic discharge in the left fronto-temporal region felt to be due to a stroke. His coumadin was adjusted upward to provide more protection against emboli and he was given Depakote to control seizure activity. He was also started on Digoxin to regulate his heart rate and Lipitor to lower his cholesterol. By the time of his discharge five days after admission, he appeared neurologically and cognitively normal.

When seen in the office in December of 2000, he had no neurologic symptoms. Examination was unremarkable including memory, thinking and language, and his pro-time was at an effective level. In April of 2001, he was asymptomatic with his pro-time in a good range. He was slightly tremulous from the Depakote, but his blood level was appropriate. EEG revealed no seizure activity and repeat MRI of the brain showed the damage from his previous strokes.

During the next two years, he continued to do well. His examinations were normal aside from mild tremulousness, with his pro-times and Depakote levels remaining therapeutic. In June of 2003, he was again admitted to the hospital in a confused state with impaired short-term memory, but no other neurologic findings. Pro-time and Depakote levels were both low, raising questions about compliance with his medications. MRI revealed multiple new areas of infarction in the left cerebellum, right parietal and right temporal lobes, right thalamus and left posterior frontal lobe. There was also significant atrophy of the left medial temporal region and hippocampus. EEG showed seizure activity in the left fronto-temporal area. His coumadin and Depakote doses were increased, then adjusted appropriately and his EEG improved a week later. However, he remained with severe short-term memory problems.

Six weeks later in the office, he was disoriented to time, did not know the president and could recall one of three objects five minutes later. Through the remainder of 2003 and all of 2004, he remained fairly stable in terms of his cognitive function, with disorientation and poor short-term memory. His MRI was unchanged and EEG showed no more seizure activity, but was slightly slow from both temporal regions. He was started on the antidepressant Lexapro by his internist with no change in his status. Aricept was also begun but did not appear to make any difference. In addition, Namenda was tried for several months then discontinued. His internist gave him Ritalin (a stimulant) as well, with no effect.

From April 2004 through April 2005, he was lost to follow-up. At the end of April 2005, he was again hospitalized with increasing confusion and multiple myoclonic jerks. He was still disoriented with extremely poor short-term memory, and his pro-time and Depakote levels were again low. When these were corrected and his myoclonic jerks controlled, he was discharged. Seen in office in May and July of 2005, there was no change in his cognitive status.

Chapter 7

LESS COMMON FORMS
OF DEMENTIA

One thing about getting old is that the past and present flow together.

May Sarton[1]

There are many different disease processes that produce dementia aside from the usual suspects we have described. In this chapter, we will briefly report on some of the less common conditions that require consideration when a person is being evaluated for cognitive dysfunction. There are numerous other afflictions responsible for dementia that are quite rare, and we will leave these to be discussed in the medical textbooks and investigative studies. The information given here is not meant to be comprehensive, but merely to help people understand the physician's deliberations when he or she assesses a patient with dementia and decides on possible treatment.

NORMAL PRESSURE HYDROCEPHALUS

Normal pressure hydrocephalus (NPH) is an enlargement of the cavities within the brain (the ventricles) not resulting from obstruction of fluid outflow or increased pressure. It was originally described by three neurologists in Boston 40 years ago,[2] and is considered a potentially reversible cause of dementia. Cerebrospinal fluid (CSF) is normally produced by structures within the ventricles called the choroid plexus, circulates through the ventricles, then over and around the brain and the spinal cord, being absorbed through formations called the arachnoid villi into the dural sinuses (large vein-like structures). In normal pressure hydrocephalus, there is difficulty absorbing CSF and the ventricles slowly dilate. While the reasons for this are not always clear, there is an association of this condition with past disorders that may have inflamed or damaged the arachnoid villi, such as subarachnoid hemorrhage (bleeding around the brain), meningitis (an infection of the spaces around the brain) and head injuries. There may be a stage in NPH where pressure in the ventricles actually increases, before there is dilatation and reduction in pressure back to normal. It is believed that stretching of certain nerve fibers in the white matter around the ventricles is responsible for the symptoms that occur. By some estimates, about a quarter million people in the United States may have normal pressure hydrocephalus.

Clinical Picture

The triad of the symptoms listed in Table 7.1 are the clinical hallmarks of normal pressure hydrocephalus, though the severity of each symptom is inconsistent from patient to patient. Classically, the problem in walking has been defined as a magnetic gait. What is meant by this is that the feet never leave the ground and the patient shuffles along with small steps. This has also been called an apractic gait, indicating that the person does not know how to walk properly, as the brain no longer directs the required sequence of moves. Weakness of the legs is usually not demonstrable. But the expected picture is not always seen and virtually any type of gait disturbance can occur, with impaired balance, freezing and falling. At times, the walking in NPH can mimic that found in Parkinson's disease. Urinary symptoms in these patients include feelings of urgency and frequency in the early stages, to frank incontinence as the disease progresses. Dementia can take any form but memory loss is usually prominent along with impaired executive function.

Diagnosis

The clinical presentation along with the findings on MRI or CT scan allow a diagnosis to be made. Parkinson's disease, Alzheimer's

Table 7.1
Characteristic Features of NPH

1) Gait Disturbances
2) Dementia
3) Urinary Incontinence

and vascular dementia, as well as normal aging need to be excluded. The typical Parkinsonian tremor is not seen, though rigidity can occur. There is also no response to the medications used in Parkinson's. The urinary incontinence prominent in NPH does not occur in Alzheimer's until later in the course of the disease. In addition, gait disturbances are not a feature of Alzheimer's until the process is far advanced. Vascular dementia may be confused more often with NPH as gait problems are frequently present. However, incontinence also tends to occur later and focal neurologic signs are often found. Some physicians unfamiliar with neurologic diagnosis may mistake normal pressure hydrocephalus for normal aging, particularly in the early stages. However, while normal older people may walk more slowly, have minor difficulty with memory and rare incontinence, the picture seen in NPH is quite different.

MRI and CT scans of the brain show the characteristic changes of enlarged ventricles disproportionate to the amount of cortical atrophy. (Enlarged ventricles are often seen as a part of cerebral atrophy in normal aging and various dementias.) Changes in the white matter around the ventricles are also found as a result of possible cerebrospinal fluid "leaking" into brain tissue. NPH cannot be a radiologic diagnosis alone, as the clinical presentation must also be compatible with the images.

Treatment

Some physicians have tried to use diuretics (water pills), particularly acetazolimide, to treat NPH in the early stages. Though occasionally a patient may respond for a short period, the results in general have not been encouraging. There is no specific medical therapy that appears to be beneficial.

The treatment currently favored involves placing a plastic tube into one of the ventricles and draining fluid into the abdominal cavity (a ventriculo-peritoneal shunt). Though television advertisements for this procedure would have us believe that severely impaired patients improve dramatically, the response is inconsistent and only a small segment of patients are truly helped. Part of the problem may be that patients are not being carefully selected, and some individuals with coexisting conditions that have damaged the brain are being shunted even though the chances of benefit are remote. Underlying Alzheimer's disease or other forms of dementia, or significant cerebrovascular disease, make it unlikely that a patient will respond to the procedure.

When a person is having major problems with brain function and is progressively deteriorating, families will grab at any life preserver offered to them, as they are reluctant to give up hope. However, in addition to being expensive, shunting is potentially dangerous, with infections not uncommon, and bleeding into or around the brain also seen. Studies have shown complication rates in the range of 13–50 percent, and the companies that make the catheters and the surgeons who perform the procedure are more enthusiastic about the results than many neurologists. A small percentage of patients with NPH are reasonable candidates for shunting and may do quite well afterward, but it is important to choose patients carefully. Lumbar punctures (spinal taps) and lumbar drainage that temporarily remove large amounts of cerebrospinal fluid from the spaces around the brain and spinal cord, and from the ventricles, may at times be a good predictor of whether a person will improve with shunting.

Though normal pressure hydrocephalus comprises a small segment of the total patients with dementia, some of them are potentially remediable. It is up to the physicians, together with the families and patients, to select those individuals who have a decent chance of getting better with a shunting procedure.

SPORADIC CREUTZFELDT- JAKOB DISEASE (CJD)

Creutzfeldt-Jakob disease is a relatively uncommon illness caused by an infectious agent called a prion, which is a misfolded form of protein able to replicate and produce severe damage to the central nervous system. It is one of a class of diseases called spongiform encephalopathies that can affect humans and various animals.[3] Unlike the usual disease processes responsible for dementia, it can be transmitted to other individuals and in some cases to other species. From the time of onset of symptoms, it progresses rapidly, with death occurring within a year.

First described in the 1920s, CJD has three forms. The sporadic disease is responsible for approximately 85–90 percent of cases. About 5–10 percent of cases are inherited and due to a mutation of the prion protein gene. Less than 1 percent of cases are transmitted iatrogenically (through medical procedures), with the use of growth hormones from cadavers, contaminated corneal transplants and dura mater (fibrous covering of the brain) transplants. Since this type of transmission was recognized, safeguards have been put into place to make this occurrence extremely unlikely. While no apparent cases have originated from blood transfusion, caution is warranted, and blood or blood products from anyone with an unusual dementia or possible CJD is to be avoided. The incidence in the United States and worldwide of the sporadic form is about one case per million population per year, with less than 300 cases of CJD reported in the United States annually.[4] There is a higher risk among the older population with a rate of 3.4 cases per million in people over age 50.

Pathology, Clinical Presentation and Diagnosis

The brain may look normal at autopsy or may show some degree of atrophy.[5] On microscopic examination however, there are characteristic "spongiform" changes in the gray matter. The term is aptly descriptive with holes of different sizes throughout the tissue giving it a sponge-like appearance. A loss of neurons also occurs. The prion that produces this disease is an abnormally folded protein resistant to sterilization because it doesn't have nucleic acids like viruses and bacteria by which they replicate themselves. It is still uncertain exactly how prions propagate. They seem to have particular affinity for the central nervous system of the animals they infect, though other tissues are also involved. At least six subtypes of the infectious prion cause CJD, and they may present in diverse ways.[6]

The diagnosis for many years was made mainly on a clinical basis, augmented by the finding of periodic sharp waves on electroencephalogram, then confirmed by brain biopsy, or at autopsy. Unfortunately, the periodic abnormalities on EEG are absent in about one-third of the cases.[7] In recent years, new tests have become available allowing a diagnosis to be verified earlier. These include cerebrospinal fluid analysis for a particular protein (14-3-3) and advances in MRI techniques.[8] High intensity signals in deep areas of the brain called the basal ganglia on MRI are felt to be fairly sensitive and specific for sporadic CJD. The use of special diffusion weighted imaging (DWI) and FLAIR studies on MRI may also be helpful, as may SPECT and PET scans.

Sporadic Creutzfeldt-Jakob disease usually occurs in people between ages 50 and 70, but can be seen at any age. Because of the diffuse involvement of the central nervous system, virtually any combination of cognitive, motor, balance, sensory and visual problems can occur. Though dementia is prominent in all cases, it may not be present initially. Eventually, all aspects of cognitive function deteriorate, with memory particularly impacted. Language is also affected, with aphasia in a large percentage of patients along with difficulty recognizing objects and understanding their meaning. Personality changes and psychiatric disturbances are frequent, ranging from depression and agitation to childlike behavior, paranoia and hallucinations.

In addition to the cognitive and psychiatric findings, myoclonic jerks are a common feature, with body twitches corresponding to the periodic discharges on the EEG. Seizures may also be seen at times. Severe imbalance (ataxia) is found as well, along with weakness on one side of the body (hemiparesis) or generalized weakness. Tone in the extremities may be increased (rigid) or decreased (flaccid) along with an increase or decrease in reflexes. This may depend on the stage of the illness and which areas of the nervous system are most involved. Difficulty with swallowing, slurring of speech and drooling occur as the disease progresses. Subjective sensory complaints are common, but objective loss is rare. Visual symptoms may include field abnormalities, cortical blindness and problems with eye movements. Sleep disturbances are also noted.

The course of the disease is extremely rapid and changes can be seen in the neurologic picture from day to day. Over a period of months, the patient may evolve from minimal symptoms to severe dementia and behavioral abnormalities: from full independence with intact strength and balance to being bedridden. Eventually, the patients become mute, unmoving and unresponsive before lapsing into coma and then dying. The total time that has elapsed is rarely more than a year, usually just months. Unfortunately, at present there is no treatment of significant benefit for this condition. Patients should be made comfortable and given therapy for symptoms such as seizures, muscle jerks, pain and so forth. Any tissues or bodily fluids should be handled carefully to be certain there is no inadvertent transmission of the disease.

VARIANT CREUTZFELDT-JAKOB DISEASE (VCJD) MAD COW DISEASE

During the early 1990s, an epidemic of bovine spongiform encephalopathy (BSE) occurred in cattle herds in Great Britain believed to be due to feeding these animals meat and bone meal containing protein from other infected ruminants. The sick cows manifested nervous or aggressive behavior, poor coordination, problems arising when lying down and abnormal postures. Death occurred after a period of two to six months. This was also a disease caused by prions, but different from those responsible for classic CJD. At first it was believed BSE would not spread to humans, but by the mid-1990s, human cases began to appear.[9] Eating contaminated beef, particularly brains or organ meats, was considered responsible. Since then, cases have been found in various countries, with Great Britain still having the largest number. Yet it remains a rare illness, with the chances of developing the disease quite small even after ingesting meat from a sick cow. At of the end of 2003, only 153 patients with vCJD had been reported throughout the world, 143 of them from Great Britain.[10] Of course, it is possible that more people will be stricken over time as the incubation period could be as long as many years or even decades. But this is somewhat unlikely since there has not been any marked increase in cases since contaminated beef was removed from the market.

In addition to the prions being different in the human cases of vCJD versus sporadic CJD, the clinical and pathologic features of the two diseases are different. According to the CDC (Centers for Disease Control and Prevention), the median age at death for classic CJD is 68 versus 28 for vCJD. The mean duration of the illness in classic CJD is 4–5 months, versus 13–14 months for vCJD. Psychiatric and behavioral symptoms are more prominent in vCJD and neurologic signs tend to be delayed compared to the classic form. Patients often complain of painful sensations (dysesthesias) in variant CJD and are less likely to have periodic discharges on their EEGs. Though the diagnosis can usually be made on clinical grounds with assistance from MRIs, autopsies or brain biopsies provide the only definitive answers. Dementia, neurologic findings and myoclonic jerks usually do not occur until later in the course of the disease.

At present, there is no treatment for vCJD except addressing the symptoms. With the risk of bovine spongiform encephalopathy now miniscule since ruminant feed for cows was discontinued, even fewer cases of vCJD will be seen in the future.

PROGRESSIVE SUPRANUCLEAR PALSY (PSP)

Progressive supranuclear palsy was originally described by three Canadian scientists in 1964 and their names are sometimes attached to the disease (Steele-Richardson-Olszewski Syndrome). This condition is often confused with Parkinson's disease, though the clinical picture is somewhat different, and occasionally with Alzheimer's. The actor Dudley Moore died with this illness in 2002. It is believed to affect about 20,000 Americans, but exact numbers are difficult to ascertain since the diagnosis is often missed. Estimates have been made of a prevalence rate of 7 per 100,000 population above 55 years of age. There have also been estimates that 4–8 percent of Parkinson's patients may actually have PSP, but this appears to be too high. The onset of the disease is usually in the sixties, but cases have been noted one to two decades earlier or later. Men appear to be affected more often than women. Although a few families have been found with several members having PSP, the vast majority of cases are sporadic and no firm genetic pattern has yet been uncovered.

Pathology and Diagnosis

There is deterioration of neurons in the basal ganglia, brain stem and cerebellum deep within the brain that control motor activity, balance and eye movements in patients with PSP. The primary motor cortex may also be affected. Neurofibrillary tangles consisting of abnormally phosphory-lated tau protein accumulate in the involved cells causing dysfunction and eventual death. This condition can be considered a tauopathy—a disease resulting from aggregates of tau protein. What initiates the process is currently unknown.

There are no definitive tests to diagnose PSP but certain findings on MRI involving the structures at the base of the brain can be supportive of the diagnosis.[11] The use of PET and SPECT scans can be helpful in excluding other entities.

Clinical Picture

The disease usually appears insidiously. The initial symptoms tend to be problems with gait and balance, along with nebulous feelings of fatigue and depression. People become unsteady on their feet, move more slowly and may suffer unexplained falls. Sometimes there is postural instability and they lurch backward or in any direction. Their entire bodies may appear stiff and ungraceful, and within three to four years they require a cane or walker. Vague changes in personality may also occur along with sleep disturbances and insomnia. Slurring of speech may be an early symptom or volume may be low with an inability to project. Twisting or tightness of the neck muscles is also seen. Unlike Parkinson's disease, tremor is uncommon, but there may be a lack of expressiveness or "masking of the face" similar to Parkinson's.

Over time, eye movements are impaired as well, which is the distinctive feature of this condition. Though the eye muscles and the nerves that enervate them are intact, the brain cells on a higher level that direct them (supranuclear) are damaged, causing the problem with movements. There is particular difficulty with downward gaze and control of the eye-lids, resulting in trouble opening the eyes, involuntary closing, frequent or diminished blinking and difficulty maintaining eye contact. Patients may complain of blurred vision or double vision, and are usually unable to follow objects on examination.

Subtle personality changes may evolve into increased irritability, peevishness and spontaneous outbursts. There may be less interest in activities that were previously pleasurable. Some patients manifest so-called pseudo-bulbar affect or emotional incontinence, with inappropriate crying or laughing. Patients with PSP also develop cognitive dysfunction, which may be mild at first but progresses to dementia as the disease advances. In general, this is not as severe as in Alzheimer's and is characterized as a subcortical dementia because the deeper structures in the brain are primarily involved. But there is slowing of mental processing, difficulty with executive function, apathy, memory impairment and diminished verbal fluency. Apathy usually is more prominent in these patients than anxiety.

Eventually, patients develop difficulty swallowing and their walking gets progressively worse, until they are relegated to wheelchairs. Urinary incontinence is another feature that appears later in the course. Though patients do not die directly because of PSP, it is usually because of its complications. With swallowing compromised, patients tend to aspirate and may choke. They are also prone to develop pneumonia due to aspiration. Severe head injuries and fractures are common as well because of the frequency of the falls.

Treatment of progressive supranuclear palsy is currently unrewarding. The use of medications, such as levodopa and dopa-agonists, effective in Parkinson's disease provide only minor and temporary benefits, if any, in PSP, affecting walking, stiffness and balance. They do not improve vision, speech or swallowing, but nevertheless should be tried. The antidepressant drugs, both SSRIs and tricyclics, are of value in some cases. Their positive effects appear to be independent of their actions as antidepressants. Botulinum toxin has been utilized to treat the eyelid spasms and closure, and neck muscle spasms with some success.

Other measures can be taken that are modestly helpful. Special glasses with prisms may lessen visual difficulties. The use of weighted appliances may reduce the propensity to fall backward. And certain exercises may diminish the stiffness in patient's joints. In addition, surgical placement of a feeding tube through the abdominal wall may be necessary when swallowing problems become advanced, alleviating the threat of aspiration. But whatever interventions are utilized, the progression of PSP continues until a complication ultimately ensues. With good care, patients may survive for many years, but the quality of life remains on a downhill course.

CORTICOBASAL DEGENERATION (CBD)

Corticobasal degeneration is a rare cause of dementia similar in many ways to PSP and also resembling Parkinson's. Its exact incidence and prevalence are uncertain. The disease is slowly progressive and eventuates in death within 10 years. Symptoms reflect a pathologic process that attacks both the cerebral cortex and deep cellular structures within the brain. These include rigidity of extremities and slowness of movements, abnormal muscle contractions with twisting of limbs called dystonia, slurred speech and tremor. Difficulty swallowing tends to be a later manifestation. Walking is invariably affected and there is often impaired coordination and lack of control over an extremity (also known as alien limb phenomenon), abnormal sensations and myoclonic jerks. Symptoms are usually more pronounced on one side of the body, slowly spreading to the other side. Language problems (aphasia) are common, involving both expression and understanding. Global cognitive impairment is also present, increasing as the disease advances: a moderate dementia without a specific pattern. Personality can be altered as well and behavioral disturbances may be seen.

CBD is also a "tauopathy" where tau protein aggregates intracellularly and forms neurofibrillary tangles. There is loss of neurons as these neurofibrillary tangles impair cellular function and eventually destroy the cells. Ballooned neurons that stain poorly may be seen, similar to those of Pick's disease. Though the findings mimic PSP, in corticobasal degeneration there is usually more cortical atrophy, particularly in the frontal and parietal lobes. To date, the cause of CBD is unknown and any genetic underpinnings have not been delineated. Diagnosis is usually made on the basis of the clinical picture, though imaging studies may provide corroborative evidence.

There is no specific treatment, but it is worth trying the medications used in Parkinson's disease which may at times be helpful. Feeding tubes to prevent aspiration are usually required in the latter stages, with choking, pneumonia or other types of infection commonly responsible for death.

HUNTINGTON'S DISEASE

Huntington's chorea, a degenerative brain disease of hereditary origin was described originally by Dr. Huntington in 1872 in a group of English immigrants to Long Island.[12] Subsequently, it was renamed Huntington's disease since cognitive and emotional symptoms may predate the chorea by many years in some cases, and the latter may occasionally not appear at all. The prevalence of Huntington's has been estimated to be about 1 per 10,000 population, suggesting that nearly 30,000 people in the United States are affected. It is transmitted as an autosomal dominant with complete penetrance. This means if a parent has the condition, there is a 50 percent chance the child will be stricken at some point, with men and women equally at risk. The genetic mutation responsible, involving IT-15 located on chromosome 4, modifies the Huntington protein normally found in all humans. The age of onset is from 15 to 65, with a mean of 35 years. Rare sporadic cases without any family history have been reported, believed to be due to spontaneous mutations.

Pathology and Diagnosis

Examination of the brains of Huntington's patients shows atrophy of the cerebral cortex, with even more pronounced atrophy in two deep structures called the caudate and putamen, along with severe loss of neurons in the involved areas. The atrophy in these structures may precede the onset of clinical symptoms and can be seen on MRI.[13] This may be a good early predictor in asymptomatic patients about the future development of Huntington's. As the disease progresses, there is even greater cell loss and atrophy throughout the brain. Intracellular and intranuclear aggregates of protein, the gene product "huntingtin," appear to be toxic to the neurons. Changes in the levels of various neurotransmitters have also been found in a number of different regions.

The diagnosis can be made if a patient has the typical symptoms and neurologic findings combined with a family history. Genetic testing showing the appropriate mutation confirms the diagnosis. Sometimes, DNA testing from an affected family member may be required if the diagnosis is uncertain. MRI and PET scans can be helpful in conjunction with the history and exam.

Clinical Picture and Treatment

The brain dysfunction in Huntington's disease results in three types of symptoms (see Table 7.2). Chorea, or involuntary, rapid movements, many with a twisting or writhing character, is the hallmark of the illness. However, it can occur in the later stages, and rarely may be minimal or absent. The uncontrollable movements may begin as tics, or repetitive twitches in different areas of the body, before progressing to full blown chorea. Eventually, there is difficulty walking, with poor balance,

Table 7.2
Clinical Picture in Huntington's Disease

1) Abnormal movements
2) Cognitive impairment
3) Psychiatric abnormalities

stumbling and falling. Coordination deteriorates and the person becomes clumsy and unable to perform tasks requiring fine movements. There is clenching of the jaw and slurring of speech. Spasms of certain muscle groups may produce a twisting of the trunk or extremities in a sustained posture called dystonia. In time, trouble with eating and swallowing also occurs.

The cognitive impairment may start as mild forgetfulness, but usually advances to a full blown dementia. All the parameters of intellectual ability become compromised, including memory, language and executive function. In addition to aphasic difficulty, the person may have problems with recognition (agnosia) and understanding how to do things (apraxia). At some point, full-time care becomes necessary.

Psychiatric abnormalities in Huntington's are varied. Depression occurs frequently and frank psychosis is not uncommon. The depression may be manifest by feelings of sadness, lack of initiative, constant fatigue, irritability and an inability to derive pleasure. Restlessness and hyperexcitability are common as well, and manic-depressive behavior may be seen. The symptoms of psychosis can include paranoia, hallucinations, delusions and aggressive behavior.

There is no specific treatment for Huntington's disease and therapy is directed toward alleviating behavioral problems and preventing complications of the illness. Antipsychotic drugs can be helpful in reducing paranoid thoughts and behavior, hallucinations, delusions and violent acts. However, dystonia can be exacerbated by some of these. Antidepressants and mood stabilizers may benefit patients who are depressed or who have bipolar dysfunction (manic-depressive). Botulinum toxin injections (botox) may be able to relieve dystonia and muscle spasms. A recent small study also suggested that cholinesterase inhibitors such as Donepezil may be of some benefit as therapy for the cognitive impairment.[14] But this needs confirmation in a larger study.

Because of the difficulty in swallowing and uncoordinated movements, choking and aspiration pneumonia are common, and often the cause of death. These risks can be lowered by serving food in small pieces, or pureeing food. Consideration may also have to be given to the use of a feeding tube. The continuous choreic movements expend a lot of energy and tend to dehydrate patients, necessitating large amounts of fluids and calories. Falling is often a danger and the use of a helmet may protect against head injuries. Pointed objects or sharp edges in the immediate environment should be removed or padded.

Work is currently proceeding on producing antibodies to fragments of the toxic protein huntingtin to see if this will be able to halt or reverse the disease process. It is, however, in an early stage of development.

The course of Huntington's is relentlessly progressive, with marked deterioration in the quality of life prior to death. The duration of the illness varies considerably and can be as long as one to three decades.

INFECTIOUS CAUSES OF DEMENTIA

Syphilis

One of the most common causes of dementia a century ago was syphilis, caused by a spirochete called Treponema pallidum. It is almost unheard of in the developed world today unless it is in conjunction with AIDS. Syphilis affecting the brain is known as general paresis and occurs as a tertiary form of the disease. This means that after the initial infection it enters a latent stage and becomes manifest decades later. The widespread use of antibiotics is the reason general paresis is so rare. Not only is the primary infection treated now, but the constant use of antibiotics for minor infections probably eliminates any surviving Treponema organisms before they can destroy brain tissue and produce dementia.

Lyme Disease

Lyme disease is also caused by a spirochete and produces an acute infection with a rash, fever, headache, malaise, achiness and fatigue responsive to various antibiotics. It can become chronic if untreated, with joint pains, fatigue and cerebral symptoms. These include difficulty concentrating, poor attention and memory problems. Full blown dementia, if it occurs, is extremely rare. However, Lyme disease should be excluded in a person with dementia in a Lyme endemic area, particularly if that individual is young, or the presentation is atypical. Blood tests for antibodies to the Lyme organism and occasionally spinal taps can be helpful in making a diagnosis. It is important to consider Lyme because the condition can potentially be improved or at least arrested with the administration of antibiotics. Unfortunately, Lyme disease has become a catch—all diagnosis being made without objective evidence of the presence of the Lyme organism, driven by certain physicians whose practice (and remuneration) focuses on Lyme disease. Because of this, many patients have been treated for months or even years with antibiotics unnecessarily.

AIDS Dementia

Infection with Human Immunodeficiency Virus (HIV) through sexual contact, or from blood or blood products, is responsible for AIDS (Acquired Immunodeficiency Syndrome). Because of the immune compromise, secondary infections can occur with unusual organisms, bacterial, fungal and viral, that may attack the nervous system and cause dementia, as well as other neurologic symptoms. But HIV itself can also involve the brain, producing cognitive impairment and ultimately dementia. The clinical picture together with the characteristic blood tests and imaging studies usually allow a diagnosis to be made.

METABOLIC PROBLEMS

Thyroid deficiency (hypothyrodism) is a reversible cause of dementia that is important to exclude in patients who have cognitive impairment. Individuals with hypothyroidism can have changes in skin and hair, weight gain, general slowing and diminished reflexes. The diagnosis can generally be made with blood tests of thyroid function.

Vitamin B 12 deficiency can be responsible for dementia alone or in combination with other neurologic symptoms (combined system disease). Blood tests can be helpful here as well. Other vitamin B deficiencies can also produce dementia and neurologic deficits, but usually as part of a picture of malnutrition or alcoholism (as discussed further in Chapter 11).

Alcohol abuse can damage neurons and result in various neurologic abnormalities including dementia, particularly in the context of vitamin deficiencies and malnutrition (as discussed further in Chapter 8).

AUTOIMMUNE DISEASES

Multiple Sclerosis

Multiple sclerosis (MS) is a disease of autoimmune origin that attacks primarily the white matter of the central nervous system and causes the loss of myelin (the white, fatty covering of the nerve fibers). Common symptoms of MS include weakness, poor balance and coordination, sensory loss and abnormal sensations, visual problems and slurred speech. However, a considerable number of MS patients also have cognitive difficulties that can progress to dementia. This is usually the result of extensive lesions throughout the brain that produce significant neurologic deficits. But occasionally, the neurologic abnormalities can be minor and the cognitive difficulties most prominent. Several immune modulating medications are available to treat MS by altering the immune response and these have had a modest effect in reducing the progression of the disease. Steroids and cancer chemotherapeutic agents have also been beneficial. The clinical presentation and imaging usually makes the diagnosis straight forward.

Lupus and Associated Disorders

The so-called collagen vascular diseases such as lupus, periarteritis nodosa, granulomatous arteritis and rheumatoid arthritis can affect the brain and produce neurologic symptoms. Focal stroke-like deficits are most common but psychiatric symptoms, even frank psychosis, and occasionally dementia can also be seen. Steroids and various combinations of drugs to reduce the immune response can be helpful in thwarting the disease process and its attacks on the brain.

Part II

LOWERING THE RISK OF DEMENTIA AND MAXIMIZING COGNITIVE FUNCTION

Chapter 8

ACCELERATED AGING, COGNITIVE RESERVE AND WHAT WE CAN'T CONTROL

Most adults draw back from the unfamiliar, perhaps because they are reluctant to demonstrate ignorance, perhaps because they have become genuinely indifferent to the interesting experiences of life.

Ashley Montagu[1]

Every single thing
Changes and is changing
Always in this world.
Yet with this same light
The moon goes on shining.

Priest Saigo[2]

ACCELERATED BRAIN AGING AND NEURONAL DAMAGE

As we have shown, human brains age at variable rates related to genetic make-up and environmental factors. To a large degree, our lifestyle choices define the nongenetic elements that affect our brains, and fortunately the majority of these are under our control. But when their potential negative aspects are not addressed, they can lead to earlier and more rapid cognitive decline than would be normally expected. If the aging process in the brain is accelerated for any reason, neurons are damaged and dementia emerges.

Diabetes

We have already mentioned diabetes as increasing the chances of brain atrophy, cognitive problems and dementia. It is a strong risk factor for Alzheimer's specifically, but even more so when combined with smoking, high blood pressure or heart disease.[3] The mechanism by which diabetes injures the brain remains a matter of debate. Some feel that heightened atherosclerosis in cerebral blood vessels may be the cause. Others feel the elevated glucose in diabetes may affect proteins and protein metabolism in the brain and that this is responsible for its malign effect. Or high glucose levels may somehow enhance inflammatory changes in brain tissue. The interrelationship between blood sugar and insulin levels may also play a role in the development of dementia, as insulin and the insulin degrading enzyme appear to affect amyloid deposition, memory and cognitive processes. Prevention of diabetes is the preferred route to take, but to minimize its impact upon the brain in those who already have it, good control is mandatory. This includes exercise, weight loss and proper diet, as well as whatever medications are necessary. Repeated and prolonged low blood sugars (hypoglycemia) from excess insulin can also result in brain injury and should be watched for carefully.

Obesity

Obesity and a sedentary lifestyle are believed to accelerate aging in all the body's organs, including the brain. Increased atherosclerosis is certainly part of the equation, but there are other mechanisms as well. Exercise has been shown to enhance cerebral circulation and raise oxygen transport to the brain, lowering the risk of both large and small strokes.[4] In animals, physical activity produces certain chemicals that encourage nerve cell growth and influence brain plasticity, promote the expansion of neural fibers and synapses and preserve the structure of brain cells.[5] (Exercise will be discussed further in the next chapter.) However, obesity alone hastens aging independent of activity. Animals on restricted caloric intake, who weigh less than their peers with free access to food, survive longer and appear healthier than their heavier companions. There have also been suggestions they perform better on tasks involving memory and cognitive function. One large study in elderly individuals that looked at the relationship between caloric intake and Alzheimer's disease found those in the quartile ingesting the most calories had an increased risk of developing Alzheimer's compared to those in the lowest quartile.[6] This was most evident in people with the APOE 4 gene. It would appear to be worthwhile for anyone at risk for dementia to avoid being overweight, given the correlation between obesity and cognitive decline.

Metabolic Syndrome

The "metabolic syndrome" also heightens brain atrophy and diminishes cognitive function. This syndrome, though somewhat controversial, has been recognized as a major risk factor for cardiovascular disease, and consists of central obesity (increased abdominal girth), high fasting blood sugars (as seen in diabetes or prediabetes), hypertension, elevated triglycerides (fats in the blood) and low HDL cholesterol (the good cholesterol). Its effects on the brain may be compounded by its diabetic component, the hypertension, and the atherosclerosis it produces in the arteries of the brain. Insulin resistance, which is characteristic of the metabolic syndrome, may appear prior to overt diabetes, and is associated with cognitive impairment.[7] All the elements listed above must be attacked early and vigorously to reduce the possible development of dementia.

Hypertension

High blood pressure alone damages the brain and speeds up the aging process. This may occur because it ravages the small blood vessels, particularly in the white matter, producing innumerable silent "ministrokes" and ischemic changes. One study showed that in healthy older patients, small increases in blood pressure over a five-year period were associated with greater brain atrophy and white matter vascular lesions.[8] The higher the systolic blood pressure in a patient at the start of the study, the more brain damage was seen. High blood pressure in midlife is a major risk factor for dementia, but plays a prominent role at any point. Even minor elevations may negatively impact the brain. Lowering the blood pressure and keeping it low should be the goal of anyone who is hypertensive or has borderline pressure. At times, this can be achieved with a change in diet and exercise, but medications are often necessary. If blood pressure is elevated in one's twenties or thirties, it may entail taking medication for 40 or 50 years. But this is certainly preferable to allowing the increased pressure to wreak havoc in the arteries of the brain over many decades. Controlling hypertension in an important step in the battle against dementia.

Hyperlipidemia

Elevated cholesterol and other lipids in the blood are risk factors for coronary artery disease and strokes. They also make a person prone to developing dementia. This would be expected simply on the basis of heightened cerebrovascular disease, but in addition, increased cholesterol levels appear to play a role in amyloid formation. Dietary restrictions, exercise and the use of statin drugs or other substances to lower cholesterol and lipids should be pursued vigorously in those whose lipid profile is abnormal.

Smoking

Smoking promotes atherosclerotic changes in the blood vessels of the brain, as well as throughout the entire body, diminishing oxygen supply and making strokes more likely. There have been some suggestions that the nicotine absorbed while smoking may protect against Alzheimer's and improve memory, but other recent studies have concluded that there is an heightened incidence of dementia and Alzheimer's in people who smoke.[9] Evidence and intuition certainly favors the latter belief. In fact, a large study has shown that in older individuals who are not demented, smoking accelerates cognitive decline, with higher rates of impairment found in those with higher cigarette pack-year exposure.[10] The negative effects of smoking far outweigh any theoretical benefits, with smoking a major accelerant of aging in general as well as for brain cells. From a health standpoint, it is better for individuals never to have smoked, but those who do should make a major effort to stop.

Alcohol and Drugs

Excessive alcohol is toxic to brain cells, producing a specific type of dementia in alcoholics called Korsakoff's syndrome (amnestic-confabulatory psychosis), often in association with thiamin, other B vitamin deficiencies and malnutrition. Though the patient is alert and aware, short-term memory is severely compromised, and the patient may make up stories to fill the gaps in memory (confabulate). It generally coexists with Wernicke's encephalopathy which causes problems with eye movements, impaired balance and confusion. Peripheral nerve damage may be present as well. The aging brain which is already plagued by vascular disease and neuronal loss may be even more susceptible to damage from alcohol and other compounds. Though small amounts of alcohol on a regular basis appear to be beneficial, there is a direct relationship between higher intake, brain atrophy and cognitive decline. One drink daily on a long-term basis may reduce the incidence of dementia, but more than two drinks a day can be injurious to the brain. Similarly, the use of street drugs can damage neurons and compromise intellectual ability. The mechanisms may be different with different substances, but all appear to have a deleterious effect on neuronal function. To protect against dementia and enhance cognition, common sense exhorts us to abstain from street drugs and immoderate use of alcohol. Unfortunately, those who start on this path usually cannot visualize the end game, or employ denial to convince themselves it will not happen to them.

Malnutrition

Though obesity and ingesting too many calories are bad for the brain, malnutrition can also cause substantial brain injury, with death of vulnerable cells, atrophy and impaired cognitive function. The brain needs certain vitamins, adequate amounts of protein and specific amino acids to work properly. If a diet is lacking in these elements, normal metabolism will be undermined and critical chemicals, including enzymes and neurotransmitters, will not be produced in sufficient amounts. Many alcoholics are also malnourished and have vitamin deficiencies, and the combination may be even more destructive to brain cells. Some older people, particularly those who live alone, do not bother to prepare meals regularly and may not have balanced diets. They may subsist on cereals, candy and cookies and other foods that assuage hunger but do not meet nutritional needs. This is even more likely if a person is depressed, where he or she may have little interest in eating, and even less in making sure the right foods are consumed. Mild cognitive impairment or early dementia are other situations where dietary deficiencies may be seen. Families, other caregivers and social agencies must be alert to these possibilities and take measures to prevent them, or correct them rapidly when they occur. In cases where intake of essential nutrients is unsatisfactory, special concentrated supplements may be helpful in keeping an elderly individual from falling into the sinkhole of malnutrition.

Stress, Anxiety and Depression

It is believed by some investigators that high stress levels over a long period are detrimental to the brain, perhaps because of the increased amount of cortisone that is generated. Studies have shown that elevation of cortisone and similar steroids impairs memory.[11] Chronic stress and anxiety may also cause structural changes within the cerebral cortex in the areas involved with memory and thinking.

As previously mentioned, depression is associated with a heightened chance of developing dementia, though some feel it may be part of the disorder itself. However, depression has been shown to be a risk factor for Alzheimer's even if the first depressive symptoms occurred more than 25 years before the dementia became manifest.[12] This certainly suggests an independent effect on the Alzheimer's process.

Sleep deprivation, induced by stress, anxiety or depression, or occurring alone, affects cognitive ability and may cause physical changes within the brain. It is easy to say we should avoid stress, anxiety and depression to protect ourselves against dementia, but finding out how to do this is another story. Aside from the issue of dementia, no one wants to feel anxious or depressed. Admitting the presence of depression or anxiety and seeking early help with these problems, can make a difference for many people.

Cardiac Surgery

Any surgical procedure in an older person is associated with a higher risk of stroke and cognitive impairment because of the possibility of a drop in blood pressure and a period of diminished oxygen supply to the brain. This can happen because of excessive bleeding or a reaction to anesthesia. But the chances of brain injury are greater in those undergoing cardiac surgery, particularly coronary artery bypass grafting (CABG) where blood flow to the heart and lungs is stopped during work on the blood vessels and a heart-lung machine is utilized to provide oxygen. Aside from a stroke rate of 3 to 4 percent, the cognitive changes were once thought to be of short duration and mainly reversible. But studies have shown a significant percentage of patients with cognitive decline five years after surgery.[13] The question raised is whether this is because of the surgery, or because of the vascular risk factors that caused blockage of the coronary arteries in the first place: hypertension, diabetes, elevated cholesterol and lipids and smoking. These other conditions may have been responsible for progressive cerebrovascular disease after the surgery and subsequent cognitive impairment from that.[14] Whatever the cause of cognitive problems afterward, cardiac surgery, indeed all surgery in older people, is not to be taken lightly because of its possible impact on the brain. Elimination of risk factors and the prevention of coronary artery disease is the best way to protect one's brain.

Head Injuries

As previously mentioned, severe or multiple head injuries at any age increase the incidence of dementia later in life. While we may be unable to influence some of the determinants of these injuries, we can significantly affect others. One of the major areas we can modify is in the use of seat belts. Having an auto accident when seat belts have not been employed makes it much more likely a head injury will occur. With the simple act of belting when we drive, we protect our brains and reduce the possibility of dementia later on. Similarly, driving while drunk or at excessive speeds exposes our brains to the risk of severe damage. Other types of perilous behavior, such as riding a bicycle without a helmet, or a motorcycle with or without a helmet, should also be avoided because of the chances of head injury. Older people with balance problems should be cautious while walking and may benefit from the use of a cane or walker if the impairment is severe enough, lessening the possibility of falling and head trauma. Physical therapy may also be helpful.

Lack of Mental Stimulation

Lack of mental stimulation may amplify aging of the brain and make cognitive impairment more probable. Keeping our minds actively engaged appears to slow intellectual decline and may even lead to improvement. When we perform complex tasks or learn new things, synapses are formed within the brain and there are more connections between neurons. It is possible this may counteract the tendency to brain atrophy that is part of aging, though mental activity has not yet been shown to produce new neurons. (This will be discussed in greater detail along with various remedial approaches in Chapter 10.)

Other Elements

There are a number of other elements that are perhaps less important, but may still accelerate brain aging and increase the incidence of dementia. One of these may be periodontal disease that affects the markers of inflammation circulating in the blood and may have an impact on the brain as well. Attention should be paid to periodontal problems and any other possible low grade infections or sources of inflammation.

It was once believed that hormone depletion in women after menopause heightened cognitive decline and that hormone replacement would protect the brain and prevent dementia. However, it has been shown that hormone replacement therapy in women does not improve cognitive function.[15] On the other hand, in men, higher testosterone levels may be associated with better cognitive performance and delay brain aging.[16] This possibility needs further investigation. (This will be discussed in Chapter 11.)

COGNITIVE RESERVE

"The cognitive reserve hypothesis suggests that there are individual differences in the ability to cope with the pathologic changes in Alzheimer disease. Innate intelligence or aspects of life experience may supply reserve in the form of a set of skills or repertoires that allow some people to cope with the pathologic changes better than others."[17] This is probably true in other forms of dementia as well. It appears that those who are most educated, have complex jobs, or function at the highest level, are less likely to develop dementia. When evaluating patients with dementia, this concept of "cognitive reserve" should be considered, particularly when the diagnosis is equivocal and the person has advanced degrees or is extremely intelligent. Some investigators believe that intelligence and education actually provide protection, though how that happens is unclear. It may simply be another example of the "use it, or lose it" phenomenon; since these people are intellectually curious and learning new things over the years, the brain's activity helps to preserve its cells in some way.

Another possibility is that those possessing great intelligence actually have a cognitive reserve lacking in most people. Because these individuals have more neurons, or more likely more synapses, due to their increased store of information and active pathways, when the brain is attacked by a dementing process, it takes longer for it to become manifest and for obvious symptoms to appear. In other words, if Alzheimer's disease begins in that person's brain, or multiple small strokes occur, dementia may not be evident for a longer time with the usual tests that are done. We must remember, if someone's mental abilities decline from an IQ of 160 to 130 due to any type of degenerative disorder, he or she is still performing at a superior level and capable of handling his or her life. Though there has been a significant loss of intellectual function, the diagnosis of dementia can not yet be applied. The individuals themselves, family members or close friends, may realize that something is wrong, but the examiners may not be able to confirm that a problem exists.

It may also be that increased mental capacity and high educational levels permit people to utilize various strategies to compensate for intellectual compromise or impaired memory, disguising their symptoms and making it more difficult to diagnose dementia. This is generally automatic behavior done at an unconscious level, allowing people to maximize their functional abilities. In this way, because of preexisting intelligence, cognitive reserve can hide an early dementia that is already present. Further brain compromise and loss of neurons may be necessary before the diagnosis can be made.

Whether the concept of cognitive reserve is valid or not, educational achievement and intelligence does make it less likely that a person will be diagnosed with dementia.

WHAT WE CAN'T CONTROL

Though there are many things we can do to prevent dementia, a number of elements are beyond our control. We must acknowledge them and work around them, directing our efforts and energy into those areas we can affect; areas that will yield results in our continuous battle to preserve cognitive function.

Genetic Make-up

We are born with a complement of genes inherited equally from our parents that cannot be altered. For some families with a history of early Alzheimer's disease, early onset of Parkinson's disease, Huntington's or other degenerative disorders, the die is cast and there is little that can be done to halt the inevitable cellular dysfunction and death that has been programmed to occur. Fortunately, though devastating for those involved, these families encompass only a small percentage of the total number of people who will develop dementia. That doesn't mean these individuals should not attempt to delay the process in every way they can, using measures that have greater success in the more common kinds of dementia. Consideration should also be given to any experimental treatment regimens being offered for familial degenerative disorders, as several genetic diseases have already been brought under control by diet and other therapies. Hopefully, in the not too distant future, gene manipulation will be able to halt or prevent these destructive processes and perhaps reverse their effects on the brain.

In terms of its widespread dissemination in the population and the heightened risk it poses for the development of Alzheimer's, the APOE 4 gene is the most important genetic factor underlying dementia. Having two copies makes the possibility of Alzheimer's even more likely than having one, but in either situation cognitive impairment and dementia is not a certainty. Having a family member with Alzheimer's should alert people to the fact they may be carrying the APOE 4 gene and are at increased risk for the disease at some point in their lives. This makes it even more critical for them to embark upon a plan of action to reduce the chances of Alzheimer's disease, and have the perseverance to adhere to their agenda.

Education and Career

As mentioned, educational attainment and high-level jobs appear to offer some protection against dementia. Unfortunately, education for the most part is something in our past, and however much regret we have about our failures and inability to go forward with our schooling, it is not a facet of our lives easily revisited. But notwithstanding our early education, there is always the opportunity for adult or continuing education that can allow us to learn again, enhancing our knowledge and thinking. (This will be discussed in Chapter 10.)

We make career choices while we are young, and though it is possible to switch to a new career later in life, it is a difficult road to tread. Where we are in our careers and the jobs we have are usually determined by where we have been before and our education. If we are unhappy in our jobs or find we are not being stimulated enough, a second career may require returning to school or obtaining additional training of some sort. This may not be feasible if we have families to support or other responsibilities to uphold. We may have to wait until retirement, or until we are laid off from a job before finding another one that is more interesting or moving to a second career.

Environmental Factors

Our living environment, where and how we were raised and the values of our community, plays a critical role in how our lives are shaped. It often determines our choice of mates and when we marry, the importance we place on education and how far we go in school, the type of job we seek and how our career evolves, the use of alcohol, drugs and cigarettes, the type of leisure activities we pursue and whether we choose to stimulate our minds, whether we exercise or are in bondage to our televisions.

Parental influences are probably the most significant part of our early environment, as much of our behavior is defined by the negative and positive reinforcement it elicits from them, which we may carry through our adult lives.

But it is not only our parents who mould us. The communities in which we grew up also write part of our story. Peer pressure may be hard to resist, whether it is in a rural town where the young people are using methamphetamine, an affluent suburb where the kids abuse alcohol or sniff glue or a ghetto where cocaine or heroin are the escape of choice. And if your friends deride learning skills as being for nerds or geeks, or educational achievement as trying to act white, can you overcome their disdain and allow your mind to grow? If the common goal is to work in a factory or at a Wal-Mart store, can you imagine yourself as a business executive, a scientist or a professional? Are we destined to labor with our bodies or our minds in order to make a living?

The adult communities where we have our homes affect the choices we make as well. If everyone around us plays golf and cards in his or her spare time, are we going to devote the necessary hours to aerobic exercise and sharpening our minds? If there is an active social life with our neighbors who eat and drink excessively, are we going to be able to restrain ourselves? If there is an emphasis on climbing the corporate ladder, large homes and material goods, are we going to remove ourselves from the rat-race? Many people do overcome the limitations placed upon them by their early environments, finding success and happiness by rejecting the values and behavior of their parents and their peers, setting and attaining unexpected goals. As an adult, we can also dismiss the mores of our neighbors and live our lives as we see fit, or even move away to a different community where peer pressures will be less.

Our past history of environmental influences also includes illnesses and various incidents, some of which seemed minor but may have injured our brains ever so slightly and thwarted learning or development. That fall from the bike when we landed on our head and were knocked out at age 8 and the concussion playing football at 16. The time we got hit in the head by the swing and had a brief seizure afterward. The flu when we were 12 and delirious for two days. The time we nearly drowned in the swimming pool and had to be revived. The bee sting with the allergic reaction where we lost consciousness. The Lyme disease that was not diagnosed for six months. These may mean nothing individually, but cumulatively may take a toll on our brains.

There are physical aspects of our environment that may also affect us, some of which we know about and others of which we may be unaware. Growing up in an old house, we may have eaten lead paint as a child which may have a residual effect on our brains. Solvents or other toxins in our drinking water may be present in small amounts but have a long-term impact upon our central nervous system. Perhaps some compound we ingested during our childhood may have damaged certain neurons and caused Parkinson's disease decades later. Living in a large city, we may have developed asthma from the particulate matter in the air, limiting physical activity later on. All of these examples are of environmental factors beyond our control that may profoundly influence our lives. But just as with our genetic make-up, we are what we are at a particular point in our lives and cannot change what already is. We can only move forward and do what we can to rewrite the script for our future.

Chapter 9

THE IMPORTANCE OF PHYSICAL ACTIVITY AND EXERCISE

Gladness of the heart is the life of a man,
And the joyfulness of a man prolongeth his days.

Apocrypha 30:22

Physical activity is essential at every stage of our lives, but perhaps even more so as we grow older. Exercise plays a significant role in reducing vascular risk factors, including blood pressure and total cholesterol, while raising good cholesterol (HDL cholesterol). Heart function and circulation are enhanced. Sexual performance is improved. The chances of diabetes and insulin resistance are lessened and inflammatory elements in the blood appear to be lowered. Because of the above effects, coronary artery disease, strokes and all-cause mortality are all greatly decreased by exercise. In addition, muscle strength and balance are improved, and the development of osteoporosis is less likely. Endorphin levels are also raised by aerobic exercise, melting away stress, depression and anxiety.

Regular exercise as we age is important as well for the overall maintenance of our bodies. When we see older people tottering along and appearing frail, much of this can be ascribed to what is called "deconditioning." Independent of strokes and neuropathies (nerve damage), people often grow weak and unsteady when they are older because they have not been exercising and using their muscles. In fact, it has been shown that nursing home residents who were bed ridden or wheelchair bound could be dramatically improved in terms of walking, strength and functional ability by exercise programs. If we keep physically active in our later years, we will be stronger, have better balance and coordination and be much less likely to become feeble shadows of the young, requiring others to meet our needs.

Only recently, however have investigators realized that physical activity also offers protection against cognitive decline and dementia, with an inverse correlation between the amount of exercise a person does and the possibility of that individual becoming demented. In other words, the more physically active you are, the less chance you have of developing dementia. Cross-sectional, prospective and retrospective epidemiological studies as well as random clinical trials have shown a strong connection between cognitive function and fitness,[1] and various measures of general physical activity and cardiopulmonary health are good predictors of cognitive ability. Studies have also reported that people who exercise regularly have faster reaction times than nonexercisers, can discriminate between multiple stimuli better, can outperform those who are not physically active on tasks involving reasoning, working memory, fluid intelligence tests and a number of other parameters. Aerobic exercise over the years is what is critical, as strength and flexibility programs have not been shown to provide any cognitive benefits for their participants. In addition, frontal lobe functions, mainly executive ability, which deteriorate disproportionately with age, have been shown to improve in individuals on a regimen of aerobic exercise, specifically walking.[2]

Though starting to exercise at an early age and maintaining this throughout life is the ideal situation and provides the most benefits, beginning a program at any age is worthwhile. Many sedentary individuals are in denial and do not want to believe that exercise is so essential, but a number of studies have confirmed this.[3] "Exercise participation has consistently emerged as a key indicator of improved cognitive function."[4]

A large Canadian investigation involving a sample of over 9,000 men and women aged 65 or older living in the community revealed a trend to increased protection against cognitive impairment, Alzheimer's disease and dementia of any type associated with regular physical activity.[5]

The Nurse's Health Study involving 18,766 women from 70 to 81 years of age showed that "higher levels of activity were associated with better cognitive performance."[6] The authors note "the apparent cognitive benefits of greater physical activity were similar in extent to being about 3 years younger in age and were associated with a 20 percent lower risk of cognitive impairment." To eliminate the possibility that preexisting intellectual decline had already reduced physical activity, the level of exercise was averaged over many years, with at least a nine year hiatus between the reports on physical activity and the evaluation of cognitive ability.

The Honolulu-Asia Aging study involving 2,257 men, age 71 to 93, who were physically capable and cognitively intact on a screening test found an increased incidence of dementia in those who walked the shortest distance daily.[7] Those who walked the most were the least likely to develop dementia. The distance the men covered was assessed from 1991 to 1993, while the evaluations for dementia were done from 1994 to 1996 and 1997 to 1999. The investigators commented that "promoting active lifestyles may have important effects on late-life cognitive function."

A recent study from Finland and Sweden reinforces the conviction that exercise is protective against dementia.[8] In this report, 1,449 persons, age 65 to 79, randomly selected from a group that had been followed since 1972 were examined in 1998 to determine if they had dementia and Alzheimer's. A significant decrease in the incidence of dementia and Alzheimer's was found in those individuals who engaged in leisure time physical activity at least twice a week in midlife, the effect even more pronounced among APOE 4 carriers. These authors note "regular physical leisure-time activity at midlife may be protective against dementia and AD later in life."

Interestingly, another report indicated that the risk of Parkinson's disease was also reduced by physical activity.[9] Previous studies in rodent models of Parkinson's disease had shown that forced exercise protected the animals from the effects of chemicals that damaged the neurons controlling motor function. This raised the question of whether people who exercised regularly would be less likely to have Parkinson's. In two very large groups (over 48,000 men and 77,000 women), it was shown that for men greater physical activity over the years was associated with a lower incidence of Parkinson's disease. The protective effect in women was less clear, though there appeared to be a reduced risk of Parkinson's that did not reach statistical significance.

There has been some thought that people with cognitive problems are less physically active because of brain dysfunction which has already begun, and that the lack of exercise is not a causative factor. However, the pattern of inactivity may precede the dementia by many years, showing that this element of lifestyle does play a role. There are also no physical reasons why those with cognitive impairment are not capable of exercising. Aerobic capacity and muscle strength has been shown to be similar in patients who are cognitively compromised and those who are normal.[10]

In addition to the reports in human subjects, animal studies have also confirmed the benefits of aerobic activity in promoting memory and learning, as well as in tasks involving executive function.[11] The critical nature of aerobic exercise as one of the pillars of a prevention program to enhance brain health and arrest cognitive decline can not be overemphasized.

MECHANISM OF ACTION

Why does exercise work to protect and improve brain function? There are a number of different possibilities and it may be that several are operative.

Reduction of Vascular Risk Factors

As was mentioned, aerobic exercise reduces vascular risk factors including diabetes, hypertension, hyperlipidemia (elevated fats and cholesterol) and coronary artery disease. The amount and intensity of exercise a person does also appears to be linked with the amount of decrease that occurs in these risk factors. This makes it less likely that a person who is physically active will have a stroke or significant cerebrovascular disease.[12] Both strokes and small vessel cerebrovascular disease heighten the chances of an individual becoming demented, most often with Alzheimer's or vascular dementia. Even a small stroke in someone with mild cognitive compromise who functioned normally may be enough to cause that individual to slip over the edge and become demented. Of course, repeated or multiple strokes greatly increase the possibility of dementia, whether or not that person had previous evidence of cognitive problems.

Another scenario is for a sedentary person to have clogging of the small blood vessels that supply the brain by atherosclerosis. Because of this, blood flow is diminished and less oxygen transferred to the tissues. As a consequence of the reduction in oxygen, neurons may function less efficiently and perhaps some of them may die. The end result is cognitive decline and eventually dementia. The unfolding of this process may take many years, or even more likely, decades. Aside from reducing atherosclerosis in the blood vessels, exercise enhances the heart's ability to pump out blood and increases circulation to the brain. A compound called nitric oxide that plays a role in controlling vascular tone is also affected by exercise and this pathway may be responsible for maintaining blood flow to the brain, carrying vital oxygen, glucose and other nutrients.

Direct Effect on the Brain

There have been a number of studies suggesting that exercise also has a direct effect on the brain, producing anatomic changes while augmenting memory. It has been claimed that physical activity may "potentially preserve neuronal structure and promote the expansion of neural fibers, synapses and capillaries."[13] When laboratory animals were placed on a program of physical exercise, those who were the most active had larger hippocampi[14] (the area of the temporal lobe involved with memory). Physical exercise seemed to enhance neurogenesis (the creation of new neurons) in the brains of young rats, as also older ones, and may moderate "age related decline in neural structures, as well as increase neuron pro-liferation."[15] This neurogenesis has been demonstrated specifically in the hippocampus and cerebral cortex. An increase in synaptic connections between neurons has been shown to occur as well. In addition, cardio-vascular fitness appeared to be correlated with the thickness of the brain's cortical tissue (the gray matter where the neurons are located). Survival of neurons also seems to be promoted by physical activity along with neuroplasticity—the ability of neurons to change and adapt to different environments and in response to various stimuli.

In mice, some specific compounds in the brain related to memory and brain function are apparently increased as the result of exercise.[16] BDNF (brain derived neurotrophic factor), a protein that enhances synapses and protects neurons from injury, was elevated in the hippocampi of mice that exercised compared to those that were sedentary. And the more the mice ran, the more BDNF was found. Those that had higher levels of this compound also performed better on tasks involving memory and learning. Animals whose memory was poor had improvement after the injection of BDNF into their brains. This suggests that BDNF may play an important role as a link between memory and exercise. The protein NGF (nerve growth factor) also rises in the brain with exercise and may provide some protection from cognitive decline. In addition, the neurotransmitter ser-otonin increases in response to exercise and may stimulate proliferation of neurons. IGF-1, a growth factor structurally similar to pro-insulin, is another substance that appears to have neuroprotective effects and is elevated by physical activity.[17] A number of genes that regulate synaptic function and neuroplasticity also seem to be impacted by exercise.

Angiogenesis, the growth of new capillaries from preexisting arteries, occurs in the brains of laboratory animals as the result of exercise, increas-ing blood flow, oxygen, glucose and other nutrients to brain tissue.[18] Seen in older rats as well as the young, this may begin days after an exercise regimen is initiated, supporting heightened neuronal activity. This mechanism of increasing blood flow to the brain could be another way aerobic exercise mitigates the cognitive decline associated with aging.

As discussed previously, some recent work raises the possibility that exercise may mobilize amyloid that has been deposited in the brains of transgenic mice with Alzheimer's changes. If this is so, exercise in humans might be able to prevent or reduce amyloid deposition in the pre-Alzheimer's stages, protecting against the development of the disease state. It is too early to know if these observations will be borne out by further studies, but it is exciting to consider this as a possible way to modify the Alzheimer's disease process.

All of the above data confirms the idea that "exercise is a powerful effector of brain physiology."[19]

Reduction of Stress and Depression

For some time, it has been known that physical activity can reduce stress and modify depression, both of which are risk factors for dementia. Though the exact manner in which this occurs is unknown, certain chemicals, such as endorphins, generated by the brain with exercise could play a role. In addition, hormones that are elevated during stress, such as cortisol, appear to block neuronal generation, and are found to be higher in some patients with Alzheimer's disease. Prolonged exposure to these hormones may damage neurons and reduce their survival, particularly in the hippocampus.[20] Studies in human volunteers injected with cortisol have found an acute deterioration in learning and recall.[21] In response to stress, neurons show dendritic (branch) atrophy and loss of spines which affects brain plasticity. BDNF, which enhances neurogenesis and neuronal proliferation, has been shown to be decreased in laboratory animals who are chronically stressed. Thus, another mechanism by which exercise could protect against dementia and cognitive decline might be by lowering stress, anxiety and depression, and stress-related hormones.

Other Pathways

Yet another possible way exercise might curb dementia could be its effect on the relationship between glucose and insulin, independent of vascular disease. Insulin, insulin growth factor, insulin degrading enzyme and elevated glucose levels in the blood appear to play a role in the development of dementia, affecting the production of beta-amyloid. Since aerobic activity decreases blood glucose, with a beneficial effect on insulin resistance and glucose intolerance, this might be the manner in which it influences dementia, similar to its protection against diabetes. Cholesterol is also an important element in the generation of beta-amyloid.

As exercise reduces blood cholesterol, it might impact beta-amyloid in the brain and thus reduce the incidence of dementia in this fashion. An additional consideration is that physical activity improves cognitive function because of its overall impact on vitality and biological aging, rather than through a specific narrow effect. People who exercise are generally healthier than their peers who do not.

It is also possible that exercise and physical activity act to protect the brain and reduce dementia by mechanisms that have not yet been elucidated. Only time will tell us for certain why it is effective. At present, animal and human studies show us that it appears to work and should be one of the basic tools we use to fight dementia. However, further large prospective studies in humans should also be done to confirm its apparent great benefits.

EXERCISE PROGRAMS TO PREVENT DEMENTIA

The questions frequently asked are—what type of exercise should I be doing, for how long and how vigorously? Recognizing that everyone's health status, physical abilities, time constraints and self-discipline are different, there are no uniform answers to these questions. A program has to be selectively tailored to meet each person's needs. In general, the more time devoted to exercise each day, the better it is for that individual. But one should strive to do at least an hour of repetitive-type aerobic activity daily, in a single time block if possible. The recommendations of the Institute of Medicine, the medical division of the National Academies support this, advising at least an hour of exercise for everyone, every day.[22] (Of course, missing a day because of time pressures, illness or injury, or other reasons, should not produce anxiety.) We should remember that there does seem to be a correlation between the amount of physical activity that is done and its protective effects against cognitive decline. But it is uncertain whether there is a point of diminishing returns. While one or two hours of exercise daily may be valuable, it is possible that five hours may confer no additional benefits. And there is always a greater potential for injury when exercising for longer periods, or at increased intensity. Though exercise physiologists suggest resting a day each week, slowing down for a day or reducing your distance may also be restorative.

In terms of what type of aerobic activity is best, it again depends on the individual. Each person should choose what is most enjoyable, easiest and most likely to be continued. It is of no value to exercise for a week or a month and then stop for one reason or another. Any aerobic exercise is good! That includes walking, running, biking, roller blading, rowing, swimming, jumping rope, using an elliptical trainer and so forth. Competitive sports, such as tennis, may be fun but with the stress involved, and the stopping and starting, are probably not as valuable as the repetitive-type activities listed above. And golf conveys no benefits unless you walk the course rapidly, perhaps carrying or pulling your bag and quickly getting off your shots. If you enjoy these sports you should continue to play, but not neglect the other kind of work outs. There are some people who find cross training pleasurable: running or walking one day, biking the next, perhaps rowing or swimming the following day. This regimen utilizes different muscles, lessening fatigue and reducing the possibility of injury. In addition, certain individuals find the different types of exercise more challenging and more interesting than the same activity every day. But whether it is one or many kinds of exercise, what is important is doing it every day. Getting into a routine and having a schedule you adhere to makes the process easier, and after awhile, for many people, it becomes almost automatic. For many older people, participating in a group while exercising makes it more enjoyable.

Ideally, you should be physically active from childhood on, so there is no need to begin an exercise regimen at some point later in life. However if you have not been exercising regularly, you should have a medical check-up before embarking on a work out program. Once you have obtained clearance, it is smart to start slowly, gradually building up the intensity and duration to where you want to be. This is not a sprint to get in shape quickly, but a long-term project that you will hopefully carry on for the rest of your life. The earlier you start, the better it is, but it is never too late to begin. There is always value from a health standpoint, and your investment of time and effort will certainly be rewarded. In terms of protection from dementia, the maximum benefit will be obtained if you are exercising regularly by your forties or fifties. (It was previously noted that obesity and a sedentary lifestyle during midlife make dementia more likely later on.) As Alzheimer's disease and vascular dementia take decades to develop, the processes responsible for producing them may be at work in your brain by this time, needing 10, 20 or 30 years to finish the job. To neutralize this ongoing attack most effectively, you should be exercising every day, even through your seventies, eighties and nineties, or as long as you possibly can. If there are limitations because of illness or some type of disability, a physician or health professional trained in this area may be able to help you devise a program suitable to your capabilities.

Walking

There are many advantages to brisk walking. It is the easiest form of exercise to start and continue; merely an elaboration of what we do normally each day. Strengthening the muscles we use walking will improve our stamina and range, help our balance and allow us to remain independent longer as we grow older. Because it is low impact and part of our daily routine, it is unlikely to cause injuries. And the equipment we need is minimal. A good pair of shoes that provides cushioning and support is essential. Proper seasonal dress should also be part of the equation. By this is meant not dressing too warmly during the summer, increasing the possibility of heat injury or dehydration, and not neglecting proper warmth on cold days in the winter, with particular protection of the hands and ears to prevent frostbite.

To go for a walk, one simply has to step out of the house and begin. That said, one should avoid areas with a lot of traffic or many cross streets which entail a lot of stopping and starting. Preferable times are early morning or early evening, away from the sun and the heat of the day. However, when walking on the road around dusk or dawn, one should wear a reflecting vest to be visible to cars, and carry a flashlight to spot any potential obstacles. Walking outside in the fresh air in the early morning can be an invigorating experience; seeing the stars flickering in the sky like distant candles, or the sun rising on a new day; watching the world shaking off its blanket of slumber and slowly coming back to life. You become one of a select group of people who have the discipline and have made the commitment to exercise at dawn, with a special feeling of control and mastery. But doing it at any time of the day or in any situation is worthwhile.

A portable radio or CD player with earphones designed to be used while exercising may make the process more tolerable for those who still maintain an aversion to physical exertion but know they must do it. (Of course, one must be cautious using earphones if walking near traffic.) Having a companion to share the miles makes walking easier for some people, with conversation accelerating the passage of time. Some walkers follow the same route every day because it is comfortable and easy, while others find it more interesting to venture frequently into new territory and vary their routes. Going to a gym and using a treadmill in the midst of other fitness acolytes is preferable for some individuals who seem to absorb energy and motivation from those around them. Using a treadmill at home, while watching the news or listening to music or books on tape, is the best environment for others.

Once you've decided on walking as your method of exercising, the questions become how much, how fast and how often. The how often is easy. Every day! There is no reason not to go for a walk daily, keeping your mind and muscles adequately tuned. After awhile, you may find that your body craves the exertion, almost like a junkie who needs a fix, and that you don't feel as well if you haven't done it. (It is probably true that there is an addictive component to aerobic exercise, perhaps because of the endorphin release.) In terms of how much and how fast, that's up to you. If more can be done, so much the better. Each individual should set a speed at which they're comfortable. Remember that this is exercise and not a stroll, so you want to get your heart rate up and be sweating: indications that you've had a work out. Covering a mile in 12 to 20 minutes is a good range for most people, with the lower end requiring more effort. Going a little faster one day and slower the next is not a bad idea, but being engaged in a continuous block of time is the best way to do it. Walking with your dog who sniffs and poops frequently should not be considered as the way to meet your exercise requirement. For most people four miles daily is a good base and generally takes about an hour. On days when you have the inclination (or more time), you can extend the distance as you desire.

Running or Jogging

Running or jogging is an excellent aerobic activity and conveys the same benefits as walking, with reduction of cardiovascular risk and protection against cognitive decline. There is a greater expenditure of energy and a greater distance can be covered in the same amount of time. On the other hand, the calories burned per mile is the same whether you are running, jogging or walking, independent of speed (a 154-pound person burns about 110 calories for every mile traveled). Unfortunately, there is a greater possibility of injury associated with running, from twisting an ankle to fracturing a bone with a fall. This is particularly so for older individuals and those who are just starting an exercise regimen. But if it is enjoyable, there is no reason not to do it. The equipment required is again minimal—good shoes and proper dress.

Biking

Biking is another attractive method of fulfilling your exercise requirements; a way that is most pleasurable for some adherents. About three miles traveled biking is equivalent to one mile walking or running. It is an activity that many have engaged in since childhood and necessitates switching from an occasional excursion to a daily work out. Having the right bike to ride can be a somewhat expensive proposition, along with a good helmet and proper clothing, but is worth the cost if it will propel you to constantly use them. It is a little more dangerous than walking or running, as a fall may cause a more severe injury. There is also the problem of avoiding traffic and dealing with cars when they intrude on your space. As we grow older and our reaction time slows and our vision is not as acute, the risks associated with biking also grow. But again, if it is satisfying and is pursued religiously, it should be continued.

Other Aerobic Activities

Roller blading, rowing, swimming, elliptical trainers, Nordic track machines and virtually every type of aerobic exercise have their own proponents. If it's enjoyable and you are willing to do it regularly, it should be the activity of choice. The main issue at times may be accessibility: having to go to a gym to use the equipment or a pool to swim. Having the machines or a lap pool in your home changes the equation. For some people this also provides the opportunity for cross training: utilizing the machines one day, walking or biking the next, then back on the machines or swimming the following day. Whatever works for you.

Because of the difficulty in getting older adults to exercise regularly in an intensive program, a Japanese group developed a regimen that was enjoyable and of mild intensity, combining club-based and home-based activities.[23] This was intended to increase participation of the elderly and combined calisthenics with singing. Cognitive function and physical abilities were measured at the start and one year later. Those who participated were found to have both improved memory and physical status, with a correlation between the two, suggesting that even a lower level of physical activity might stem cognitive decline. This was hypothesized to also be of potential benefit in those with mild cognitive impairment.

I have not mentioned weight work or stretching as playing a role in preserving cognitive function, and indeed they don't. However, stretching is important for the health of our musculo-skeletal apparatus—keeping our muscles, tendons and joints in good shape to allow us to continue aerobic activity. So these routines should not be overlooked. Likewise, weight work develops muscle strength and reinforces bone health. So this type of regimen should not be neglected.

Most people don't like to exercise. They see it as unpleasant work and time consuming to boot, when time for many individuals is at a premium. In addition, in many advanced societies, people are unused to physical exertion and derive no enjoyment from it. They find the sweating, the muscle aching and occasional discomfort off-putting and do whatever they can to avoid it, aside from competitive games or sports. Some highly educated individuals who barely move in a temperature controlled office all day even see physical activity as beneath them; more in the realm of blue-collar workers who can't use their minds to earn a living and have to sweat to make a buck. This has to change. There is no dichotomy, no either-or rule that forces a person to use either his or her mind or body. In fact, it is important that we exercise both our minds and our bodies regularly, and keep each apparatus finely tuned and in the best shape.

The emotional baggage and psychology associated with exertion and physical activity in developed societies must be overcome. We all have to convince ourselves of exercise's value so that we want to do it and it becomes an automatic part of our daily routine. We have to view it through a lens that emphasizes its benefits and pleasures; not just in halting cognitive decline but the way it can relax us and improve our physical prowess; the way it reduces heart disease and strokes, diabetes and osteo-porosis; the way it can increase our longevity and enhance our quality of life. Of course, many people already know that it's good for them but perceive it as work and don't want to expend the effort to exercise. Some are fatalistic and won't believe they can control their lives or change what lies ahead, no matter what they do. And other sedentary individuals are in denial, like smokers, and feel that the illnesses associated with physical inactivity will not strike them, so it's unnecessary to change their tunes and start exercising.

Certain images embedded in my mind promote the essentiality of exer-cise. On a visit to Ferrara, Italy, a few years ago, I was struck by the legions of bikers everywhere I went in the city. Even old women in their seventies and eighties pedaled to and from the market, with fresh loaves of bread sticking out of their baskets which were undoubtably also filled with pasta and fresh produce. And almost no one was fat. The food was wonderful and plentiful, and eating was a joy, but the activities of the day kept people's weight in check. In other cities, people were walking as well as biking, and physical activity was accepted as a normal part of life. Though everyone was eating pasta and drinking wine, obesity was uncommon.

In Vietnam, there were also hordes of bikers everywhere. Farmers would walk into the cities in the early morning with baskets on long poles, or ride bikes with enormous baskets carrying their produce to the local markets for sale. If not on a bike, walking was the normal way to get around for people of all ages. And almost no one was overweight.

Then there were the National Geographic television specials focusing on the mountain villages in the Caucasus, where everyone walked and worked, treading over the steep mountain trails every day, toiling in the fields or in some job that required physical exertion. The men and women were particularly long-lived, seemingly functional and cognitively intact. And they were all fairly thin. Most people survived into their nineties or were centenarians, with some as old as 120 or more.

These images are all of people who are physically active and not obese, where exertion and exercise are ingrained in their lives. Interestingly, in the United States, there are less obese people living in those cities with good transportation systems than in the suburbs. In the cities, people generally can't use cars to get around, but walk or take public transportation. And when using buses or subways to travel long distances, they still have to walk to and from these fixed routes. Overall, they are in better physical shape than their neighbors in the towns and villages outside the cities.

In the suburbs people seem to loathe walking. They drive everywhere, since it is easy to park and access their cars. Even on short trips of less than half a mile, they are likely to hop into their automobiles rather than walk. Though there are some individuals devoted to physical fitness in both the cities and the suburbs, the vast majority in the suburbs won't walk simply because they don't have to. In the cities, people have little choice. The rural regions present a mixed picture. Though the inhabitants usually drive everywhere since the distances to be traversed generally preclude walking, they are more likely to be engaged in work requiring physical exertion. Thus, they may be in better shape than their comrades in the suburbs. But the cities, suburbs and rural areas all have too many obese and overweight people who lead sedentary lives and eat the wrong foods. It can't remain this way. Everyone has to get the message that exercise is important and what you eat and how much you eat is critical. I am not just talking about how long people live, but the quality of their lives and what they can do while they are alive.

We all have the potential to live healthy lives with our brains functioning at a high level if we do the right things. I recently attended my fiftieth high school reunion and was amazed at the different ways my classmates had aged. Unfortunately, time had not been kind to many of them. A large proportion were overweight and many were limited by various physical ailments. And I assume, this was a select group: the ones who were relatively intact and able to get to the reunion. In speaking to a number of them, I found very few who exercised regularly and vigorously. (I did not question them about their eating habits.) Most of them had previously done sedentary work of one sort or another and were now retired, though a number of the women had raised children and not worked. They were people in their mid to late sixties, who could have achieved a large degree of control over their lives, but perhaps had not had the knowledge, interest or discipline to maintain an exercise program over the years. I hate to think how many of them will be attacked by strokes and dementia in the next two decades.

In our current information age, the vast majority of us have jobs that are physically undemanding, sitting at desks and working at computers. We go out for lunch at nearby fast food establishments. Then after more sitting at our desks, we pop into our cars to go home, or get where we want: a few drinks at the local watering hole, or a large, rich meal at a restaurant. It wasn't like this a century ago. People may have died earlier of infectious diseases such as TB or pneumonia, but they were physically more active and perhaps healthier. There was not as much dementia, perhaps because people did not live as long, or maybe because it was not recognized. Older people who were demented were called senile and it was considered a normal part of aging. We now know it is not normal and there are steps we can take to prevent it. But we have to get off our behinds and play a diligent role in doing what is required.

The psychological impediments associated with physical activity in America and other industrialized countries have to be removed. We have to stop looking at exercise as a chore and imbue it with positive attributes, knowing that it is a necessity. If it is not pleasurable, we have to play mind games with ourselves to make it seem pleasurable. Perhaps self-competition can be helpful in that regard as we push ourselves to go a little bit further, or a little bit faster than we had first envisioned. After setting goals that we wish to attain, we can then compete with ourselves to reach or even surpass these goals. By competing with ourselves, we can make the process more interesting, yet not feel the pressure of pitting ourselves against another person with the label of winner or loser.

Integrative Exercise

In addition to any formal exercising we do, we should also try to increase overall physical activity in our lives. Any small incremental moments of exertion may be valuable over time. By this I mean climbing the stairs whenever reasonable instead of taking an elevator. Walking or riding our bikes rather than using cars to do our errands, such as picking up groceries or the newspaper or whatever. Mowing the lawn by hand, or shoveling snow, rather than paying a local teenager (if you can find one willing) to do the job. This type of activity has been labeled "integrative exercise" by fitness professionals because it incorporates exercise into the tasks of everyday living.[24] That said, make sure you have medical clearance before performing vigorous tasks if you haven't done them regularly. All of these activities help to keep us physically fit and make it more likely that we will be able to maintain our independence as we grow older. The more we do, the more we are able to do. Use it or lose it. And keeping our bodies going also helps to prevent the deterioration of our minds. Exercise empowers people in many ways, allowing them to take control of their lives. Individuals who exercise look better and feel better about themselves. They are generally more productive, with more energy and stamina than their peers. In fact, some planners designing communities for the future are considering ways to ensure that walking and other physical activities will become part of the daily routine.

There was a time when physical exertion was not denigrated: when people had to use their muscles as well as their minds to sustain themselves. With the technological advances of the past century, it is now possible earn a living spending every day ensconced in a comfortable chair. This is not the way we were meant to exist. To maximize the quality of our lives, reduce illness and cognitive decline, we must adopt the mind-set of the past and push ourselves to be physically active.

Chapter 10

THE NEED FOR
COGNITIVE STIMULATION
AND SOCIALIZATION

From memory, experience is produced in man.

Aristotle—Metaphysics[1]

Anyone who stops learning is old, whether 20 or 80. Anyone who keeps learning stays young.

Henry Ford[2]

Common sense tells us that to stay the hand of dementia, we must keep our minds active by learning, analyzing and reasoning as we grow older. However, there is more than common sense behind this directive, as multiple studies and reams of data lend support. Intellectual stimulation is as critical for us as exercise is in trying to prevent cognitive decline, another example of the "use it or lose it" doctrine. And like physical activity, where we climb a flight of stairs instead of taking the elevator, we should try to incorporate cognitive activity into our daily lives, using our brains in small ways and for small tasks, as well as with larger projects. Of course, learning and constantly challenging our minds with new concepts and new queries should be a lifetime endeavor of inherent value, and not done simply because it will benefit us in the future. But it is undoubtably of long-term value in helping to preserve our brains.

To protect us from the tide of cognitive decline that so frequently accompanies aging, we each need to build our own series of dikes and levees, fashioned out of knowledge and experience. Cognitive reserve was mentioned in Chapter 8; the idea that extremely intelligent or highly educated individuals may have some extra protection against dementia. Perhaps through learning and intellectual stimulation, each of us can construct our own reservoir of cognitive resources we can draw upon if required in the future. I like to use the term "cognitive engagement" to describe what we have to do. We have to be alert and attentive to the world around us and people around us, questioning, commenting and seeking to understand why things are the way they are. The more we do this, the better off we will be. Curiosity may have killed a cat, but it may also create new synapses for us and help to ensure brain health. We need to be participants in the great game of life, rather than just passive observers.

Some social analysts have divided life into three stages—education, work and leisure. This arbitrary separation should be eliminated, for it is not good for any of us. Though perhaps at different ratios, there needs to be a mixture of these three elements throughout our lives to make them exciting and pleasurable, and to keep our minds functioning at peak efficiency.

Studies in aged beagle dogs (8–12 years old) have shown that an enriched environment that provided cognitive stimulation was able to enhance learning and slow cognitive decline.[3] In other words, you could teach an old dog new tricks. The enriched environment included being housed with other dogs, exercising for brief periods twice a week, being given sets of toys that were alternated each week and testing in discrimination problems which required some mental work. After two years, the dogs having the enriched environment were found to have greater cognitive abilities than those lacking this stimulation. Cognitive function was measured by the manner in which tasks were performed that required new learning. Spatial memory was also improved. A special diet fortified with antioxidants combined with behavioral enrichment raised the abilities of these older dogs even more.

Similar results were obtained in transgenic mice who are prone to develop Alzheimer's-like changes in their brains.[4] One group was maintained in standard shoe-box-style mouse cages, while the other half was placed in large enrichment cages that contained exercise wheels, cardboard boxes, nesting material and a large social structure. Cognitive testing was done after 5–7 months followed by biochemical and histological assessment. The group from the enriched environment was found to perform significantly better on cognitive testing than those mice in standard housing, showing that the expected learning and memory deficits could be prevented.

A number of studies in humans have also found that cognitive stimulation reduces the risk of developing dementia.[5] Cognitive engagement was verified through analysis of activities in which the subjects were involved and correlated with the subsequent incidence of dementia in the different groups.

One study which took place between 1994 and 2001, followed 801 older Catholic nuns, priests and brothers throughout the United States who on testing were intact initially.[6] Their participation in activities that required information processing was then assessed at baseline. These included reading newspapers, reading magazines, listening to television and radio, playing cards or checkers, doing crossword puzzles and going to museums. Point scores were assigned for frequency of these activities and a composite measure was calculated. Subsequently, extensive yearly evaluations of cognitive function were performed, with a mean follow-up of 4.5 years. During this period, 111 persons developed Alzheimer's disease. A reduction in intellectual decline, and particularly in working memory, perceptual speed and episodic memory, was associated with higher levels of cognitive activity. Those individuals with the highest levels (90th percentile) were 47 percent less likely to develop Alzheimer's disease than those with infrequent activity (10th percentile). This data suggested a diminished risk of Alzheimer's in older people who maintain mental stimulation. The authors hypothesize that cognitive activity may be protective against Alzheimer's, or that it may bolster processing skills, such as working memory and perceptual speed which could compensate for age related decline in other cognitive domains.

Another study looked at the relationship between leisure activities and the risk of dementia in 469 people older than 75 who resided in the community and were cognitively normal at baseline.[7] During a median follow-up of 5.1 years, 124 of the subjects developed dementia. Alzheimer's was diagnosed in 61, vascular dementia in 30, mixed dementia in 25 and other types in 8. Higher levels of participation in certain leisure activities were found to be associated with a lower risk of dementia, including reading, playing board games, playing musical instruments and dancing. Those individuals with scores in the highest third on the cognitive activity scale had a 63 percent lower risk of dementia than those ranked in the lowest third. This appeared to be true for both Alzheimer's and vascular dementia. The authors believe that involvement in cognitive activities is linked to slower rates of cognitive decline, especially episodic memory. They theorize that these leisure activities might increase cognitive reserve in participants, delaying the presentation of dementia, or could affect the disease processes in some way during the preclinical phases.

In yet another report, a large group of people in Chicago who were 65 and older (6,158) were given brief performance tests of episodic memory, perceptual speed and global cognition, and were interviewed regarding frequency of participation in various cognitive and physical activities.[8] The cognitive efforts were similar to those previously described. A random sample of those free of Alzheimer's disease at baseline (835) then had evaluations after an average of 4.1 years. One-hundred-and-thirty-nine of these people were diagnosed at that point as having Alzheimer's. The investigators found that individuals with the highest levels of cognitive activity (90th percentile) were half as likely to develop Alzheimer's than those with the lowest levels (10th percentile). The authors hypothesize that the lower incidence of Alzheimer's associated with higher educational achievement and complex occupations may be because these individuals are involved in more cognitively stimulating activities than less educated persons and those with less demanding jobs. They also believe that frequent cognitive activity enhances the abilities of those involved in these programs, and so more Alzheimer's pathology is needed for intellectual decline to become manifest.

A fourth investigation followed 1772 individuals, 65 and older, living in the community in northern Manhattan, who were nondemented at baseline, and assessed their leisure activities.[9] They were then evaluated for the development of dementia for up to seven years, with a mean of almost three years. Two hundred and seven of these subjects became demented during this period. Those individuals with high participation in leisure activities, such as reading magazines or newspapers, visiting friends or relatives, going out to the movies or restaurants and walking for pleasure or going on excursions, had a decreased risk of dementia. The individuals who read newspapers or magazines, played cards or games, or went to classes, had the lowest relative risk . But there was a reduced risk as well in those who participated in social and physical activities. Even after controlling for ethnic group, education and occupation, people with high leisure activity had 38 percent less risk of becoming demented. These investigators felt there was a small possibility that reduced cognitive activities could have been an indication of early dementia, but believed it was unlikely. The importance of socialization as well as cognitive activities to lower the risk of dementia was emphasized. The authors conclude "that interventions that enhance life experiences and activities might reduce the risk of developing dementia."

The above studies and others have shown that in addition to continued learning and cognitive stimulation as we age, we also have to be engaged socially and interact with other people: friends, family, acquaintances and even strangers. Reclusive behavior and lack of social contact tends to be a prescription for cognitive decline, while socialization has been shown to be an important element in protecting against dementia.

Mechanism of Action

We have described a number of reports in both animals and humans showing positive effects of cognitive stimulation on the brain with a reduction in intellectual decline. How this occurs has not been fully elucidated, but we can exclude some of the hypotheses entertained for exercise. Cognitive stimulation does not affect vascular risk factors such as hypertension, diabetes, elevated lipids and cholesterol and atherosclerosis. It does not lower stress levels, and in some instances, could theoretically increase stress and anxiety. Unfortunately, for cognitive stimulation we do not have as much animal data as we have for exercise, showing specific structural changes in the brain and the production of specific substances that appear to be protective. Though there are reports noting alterations in the brains of animals in "enriched environments," the hypotheses regarding the way cognitive stimulation might protect against dementia must be considered to be speculative. Part of the problem is that some physical activity is usually included in these enriched environments, and separating out the effects of pure cognitive stimulation on the brain is more difficult.

Aside from changes in the blood vessels, the modifications in the brain presumed to occur with cognitive stimulation are similar to those noted with exercise. Brain plasticity and remodeling of neuronal circuitry appear to be promoted by behavioral enrichment (which may include some exercise).[10] Neurogenesis (the creation of new neurons) may be encouraged by cognitive activities, possibly in areas of the brain related to memory and learning such as the hippocampus and medial temporal lobe. Chronic neuronal activation may be seen in association with heightened brain work, along with an increase in blood flow, glucose and oxygen metabolism in particular regions of the brain.[11] Certainly, increased generation of synapses must take place as is found with any experiential stimulus. "Learning selectively enhances synaptogenesis."[12] This physiologic process eventuates in increased synaptic density in the neocortex, the thinking part of the brain, and the more cognitive activity, the more synapses might be expected to be formed. (This, of course, may be part of the construct addressed in a previous chapter regarding the loss of intelligence with aging, as wisdom is acquired.) Though elevated levels of neurotransmitters can be surmised to occur with the increase in synapses, we do not know if compounds like BDNF and NGF also rise. But more synapses and neurogenesis should provide some protection against the Alzheimer's process and other dementias.

It is not clear why socialization should reduce the risk of developing dementia, but it does seem to play a role in both humans and animals. Possibly, its effect could be mediated through a decrease in stress and depression, and hormonal changes that may accompany this. A number of strategies utilized to foster cognitive stimulation also involve social contact to a greater or lesser degree.

In animal and human studies, both cognitive stimulation and socialization appear to provide some protection against cognitive decline and dementia. However, more and larger studies are necessary to verify the work that has been done, and prove their benefits without question.

COGNITIVE ACTIVITIES

The activities discussed in the reminder of this chapter are intellectually stimulating in various ways. They require cognitive engagement of differing degrees and are enriching experientially. Though it is likely that they are beneficial in delaying or preventing cognitive decline and dementia, there is no hard evidence to support any specific activity being effective. Even then, people who are complacent and neglect these activities and mind enhancement as they grow older, do so at their own peril. It should also be understood that it is impossible for anyone to embrace all the forms of cognitive stimulation being described. As with exercise, people should focus on those they find enjoyable and are likely to continue.

Work

For many of us, work is the major source of intellectual challenge in our lives, as well as a place of social contact. Of course, the amount of stimulation we derive from work depends on the nature of our jobs. Manual labor that does not require the use of our minds, or repetitive boring tasks that fill the day, are of little value in staying cognitive decline or dementia. On the other hand, in addition to academic and scientific positions, many executive, professional, supervisory, service or sales jobs demand learning, innovation and creativity to varying degrees and meet the criteria for cognitive stimulation. Even if 90 percent of a job is routine, the other interesting 10 percent may serve to stretch the boundaries of our minds.

Yet for many individuals, retirement looms on the horizon or has already happened: the elephant always is with us in the room. This may be because of corporate, academic or government rules, or self-generated at a particular age, even though we are physically healthy and mentally sharp, and able to perform our jobs quite well. A half century ago, when most people were engaged in physically strenuous work throughout their lives, the breakdown of their bodies mandated retirement, usually by age 65. In addition, average survival was only into the late sixties, allowing only a few years of leisure before death intervened.

Currently, the majority of our populace toils with the minds rather than the bodies, perhaps sitting at a computer much of the day, to the point that physical activity has to be urged upon these people by their physicians and public health authorities. And average survival now is at least into the late seventies and early eighties, but even greater for those people who have already reached their sixties. A person who is 65 is likely to be around at age 85 or 90. This means, of course, that these individuals may well have another 20 to 30 years on their hands. How do we fill this time in ways that will hone the keenness of our minds? Golf and fishing are not the answer, though periods of relaxation are not to be derided. For many people, continuing to work an extra 5 or 10 years, or even longer, may be the best way to keep their brains functioning at a high level. When I am asked, I advise my patients to keep working, unless they have planned for other activities that are mentally stimulating. However, they should retire if the job is too stressful, or uninteresting.

Continuing to work instead of retiring may require us to rethink the accepted progression of life. Many retirees are not really happy during these so-called golden years and fondly remember the time they were still employed. Some individuals have their identities linked to their jobs and are depressed when they retire, having derived feelings of self-esteem and relevance from their work. After short periods of retirement, innumerable people try to return to their previous occupations, though most of them are unable to do so. Some crave work mainly for financial reasons, having miscalculated their needs, and find only low-skilled jobs. But others may be bored in retirement and seek the stimulation and camaraderie they recently had. This is not to say that work is a panacea, as stress, competition and personality conflicts can be problems. However, older workers are generally less competitive and not looking to advance within the corporate structure. They are usually team players, compassionate and understanding, and helpful to younger co-workers. In many ways, they are excellent employees.

Corporations will also have to change to accommodate older workers, but this may already be happening. With the baby boomers approaching retirement age, many companies are finding themselves short of skilled workers, knowledgeable employees and good salespeople, with no ready replacements. To keep older employees on board, they are willing to alter the rules and make concessions. This can be beneficial to both the individual workers and the companies. Though people may desire to continue working, they may not want to do so full-time, with commuting and whatever else is entailed. Instead, three times a week may be just right for someone. Or more flexible hours, perhaps starting at 10 and ending at 4. Or doing more work at home. Or more teleconferencing rather than traveling. For most companies, these types of adjustments can easily be made.

Some corporations have been reluctant to hire older workers because of false perceptions that need to be dispelled. One is that older people can't learn new technology and new ways of doing things. This is totally untrue. Older individuals can learn quite well, though it may take them somewhat longer. And they are able to retain any information they have learned. Another canard is that they cannot be as productive because they work more slowly. While it may be true that they are slower with certain activities, they are also more careful and make fewer mistakes, and thus can be just as productive as their younger colleagues. They are also more reliable, with less absenteeism and problems related to alcohol or drug abuse.

If their employers are unwilling to allow older individuals to continue in their previous positions, a number of options are open if they wish to keep working. They can look for a job doing similar work with another company. Or they can become self-employed or perhaps consultants in the same field. Or they can try something completely different: a job in a different field or a second career. For an older person to start a new career, or a new job later in life may be stressful, but is often cognitively stimulating, requiring learning new routines and new materials. Work is certainly one pathway to an agile, responsive mind.

(State and federal legislation will also be necessary in the future in recognition of people living longer and wanting to work longer. Employment laws and Social Security laws will have to be changed to fit with the new reality.)

Volunteering

Volunteering is a major avocation for many older people, a win-win situation, with both the organizations and volunteers benefitting. In addition to the activity itself and any intellectual energy that might be generated, there is also the opportunity to interact with other people. The type of organization chosen and the kind of position sought depends on the individual's interests and capabilities. Although performing some repetitive or menial tasks may be necessary, the more desirable jobs require thought, deliberation, problem-solving or decision-making. But sometimes, as with regular employment, one has to start at a lower level to prove competence and reliability before advancing to a more responsible post. The most common types of not-for-profit organizations seeking volunteers include religious, health care, educational, legal, senior-focused and general charitable organizations. Political groups, either issue-oriented or party derived, local or national, are also always looking for volunteer help.

Political organizations may use volunteers for fund-raising, voter registration, canvassing, get-out-the-vote efforts, disbursing information, producing or distributing campaign material, in an educational role, etc. In local campaigns or with single issue groups, there may be great opportunities for hands-on involvement and decision-making. While acting as a foot-soldier and sending out campaign literature promoting your political convictions may help your cause, it may not provide the kind of mental stimulation you need. Interesting work that keeps your mind churning should be the goal with any volunteering.

Assisting educational organizations or working in schools can be particularly rewarding. For example, one can mentor a child on a one-to-one basis. An older person can also function as a teacher's aide, or help with a specific subject in which he or she is proficient. Or the older person can tutor a child in or out of school. (It is also possible to take up teaching as a second career even later in life.) Providing administrative assistance for a school or a school district is another possibility, working with the PTA, raising funds for a special project, lobbying local governments or the state legislature about educational content or funds.

Health care is another area where volunteers play a major role. Within a hospital, a person can assist with administrative work, ferry patients about, help with educational tasks, work with bereavement groups, provide support to families when patients are in critical care, run the hospital gift shop or raise funds. There are also opportunities to volunteer with many disease-oriented charities, such as the Alzheimer's Association, the American Cancer Society, the American Heart Association, the National Stroke Association and innumerable other groups.

Working with a local church, synagogue or mosque in various positions can be cognitively stimulating while supporting your religious beliefs. Teaching the bible or aspects of the religion, helping administratively, working with youth groups, raising funds are all possibilities. People also may find involvement with the homeless rewarding, as also soup kitchens, or outreach programs, or missionary work. Some prefer to volunteer with national religious organizations, or devote their time to specific issues of concern to their religion.

Legal groups may focus on civil rights, perceived inequities in the justice system, helping victims of crime, rehabilitating felons, encroachment of government on individual rights, court reform, advocates for children and many other aspects of the legal system, both criminal and civil. Again, finding the proper organization and job depends on your needs, interests, experience and abilities.

There are many senior-oriented groups on a local and national basis that are always looking for assistance. These would include senior centers with on-site and off-site programs, Meals on Wheels, organizations that provide transportation to seniors who can't drive for medical appointments, companionship, help with shopping and various other services. On a national level, there is AARP in addition to a number of different advocacy groups.

Charitable organizations that welcome volunteers are limitless in number, type and scope, supporting museums, theaters, orchestras and other cultural institutions, famine relief, promoting peace, aiding with disasters, etc. In this realm, there are innumerable opportunities for volunteers.

Education

Furthering one's education is always a worthy goal, no less so as one ages. Constantly absorbing new information or learning new techniques is a way to expand our minds, forming new synapses between neurons and possibly even generating new neurons. There are many routes that education and learning can take, all of which have value in combating cognitive decline. First, there is the concept of self-teaching: instilling knowledge through one's own efforts by reading, studying and mastering without outside assistance. Hopefully, there is enough curiosity and interest in most of us to partake of at least some degree of self-teaching on a regular basis. Without a desire to know, all may be lost, as I can visualize brains steadily shrinking and neurons dying.

There is also the road of formal classes through universities, community colleges, high schools or senior centers. These can be audited or taken for credit, attending and listening to lectures, reading assignments, writing papers and perhaps even taking tests. Many cities and towns have a full schedule of continuing education classes for people of all ages, where virtually any subject can be found. A number of universities have special programs for alumni or individuals in neighboring areas. Some of these institutions have even developed residential communities for older people who want to participate in lifelong learning and are willing to center their lives around an academic setting. There are also stand alone lectures of various kinds that can be helpful in gaining an understanding of different topics.

In addition, there are Elderhostels that provide a plethora of subjects in numerous locations for defined periods, often combining learning with travel. The explosive growth of this concept is a measure of how hungry older people are for knowledge and learning. Over a period of about a quarter century, Elderhostel has gone from a few courses and 240 participants at a few New England colleges to 10,000 courses with more than 300,000 attendees in traditional and more esoteric sites.[13] Without doubt, these will continue to expand.

Computers and the Internet

With the widespread availability and affordability of this technology, there is no excuse for anyone not to be computer savvy. In fact, to be considered literate and relevant in this day and age, a person must be able to use a computer and navigate the Internet. Some older individuals who did not grow up with computers may be "technophobic," but with the help of professionals (such as high school students), and adequate training and supervision, this fear can be overcome. To avail ourselves of all the opportunities the Internet provides, broadband connectivity is also to be encouraged.

In terms of mental stimulation, the main advantage of computers and the Internet is rapid access to a storehouse of information on any subject. This is always at our fingertips through the use of various search engines and there is no question that needs go unanswered. Trying to remember some past event? It's right there for us. Debating some issue with a friend? It's easy to discover what actually happened. In addition to retrieving general information, we can focus on specific subjects and learn all about them. We can take classes online as well, read newspapers online and see news programs online.

Computers have also encouraged communication with other people through e-mail and instant messaging. Internet telephony is in the process of expanding and webcams allow us to talk to distant friends face to face. There are chat rooms, blogs and web sites to give us insights into other views. Dialogues and discussions can also be set up with other people, and there are games of various sorts waiting to be played: chess with a partner, or solitaire with the computer itself. And there are online auction sites that can add excitement to our lives. Because there is so much that is intriguing on the Internet, one has to be cautious about becoming addicted to this medium and not maintaining a balance in life. But using it properly will certainly keep us cognitively engaged.

Games and Puzzles

Games and puzzles interest, and are intellectually challenging for many people. We are not speaking of one arm bandits that are mind numbing, or bingo that requires minimal brain utilization, but games such as scrabble, chess, checkers, bridge and various other card games or board games that are more complex. Those that utilize concentration, memory, analysis and strategy are the ones most valuable in terms of cognitive function. Crossword puzzles, other types of word games and numerical puzzles are stimulative as well, and jigsaw puzzles reinforce visuo-spatial skills. Playing games with other people is even better than competing with a computer, as social interaction itself also helps to delay cognitive decline.

Creative Endeavors

Many individuals have nascent creative urges that cannot be fulfilled when they are younger because of employment and family commitments. As we grow older, particularly after retirement, we have more time on our hands and can indulge some of these fantasies of our youth, allowing our talents to flower. Various creative endeavors not only satisfy suppressed desires that some of us have, but are also a form of beneficial mental activity. Fields of art that attract people include painting, sculpting, photography, pottery, jewelry making and weaving. Knitting can also be creative if you do more than just follow instructions. In our digital age, some people even opt for film making in later life. Many cities and towns have classes through continuing education at the high schools, community colleges or senior centers to teach the fundamentals of the creative arts, or to provide ongoing instruction.

Writing, either fiction or nonfiction, is another expressive forum for people in their later years, which can be burnished by classes, with critiques from teachers and other students. This can be painful at times, but like a plant requiring pruning, does aid in growth.

People with previously suppressed musical talents can opt to develop them further as they grow older. The venues may include singing in a choir, a barbershop quartet or other groups, or by way of individual instruction. Learning to play the piano or other musical instruments can also be appealing, as can be participation in an orchestra or band. Dancing is a way for people to combine movement with music, and is another mechanism for creativity. Most are interested mainly in ballroom, line or square dancing, but some try ballet or jazz dancing.

The theater provides opportunities in many different areas to harness abilities previously undiscovered or underutilized. Acting, directing, set design, producing or even play writing allow individuals to express themselves in new ways. There are community theater groups in most cities and towns always looking for new members. Participating in an organization with a common goal is an additional benefit. One does not have to be a John Barrymore or Helen Hayes to derive enjoyment and satisfaction from working in the theater or theatrical productions. There are also discussion groups focused on theater, and clubs that travel to different cities to see plays.

Reading

Reading of any sort can provide some intellectual growth, but more difficult material requiring concentration and analysis is of greater value. Book clubs and discussion groups with interpretation and debate enhance the benefits even more. In addition to books, people should read the newspapers and news magazines regularly. Being able to discuss current events regarding national, international and local happenings helps with social interactions, apart from being stimulative.

Travel

Travel to new places within and outside the country has always been felt to be a broadening experience and this is just as true when we are older. We are speaking of more than just visiting the grandchildren in

California during vacations, or a cruise to the Carribean. Having contact with new cultures in foreign lands and learning about history, geography and nature in different regions can be eye opening for us. Even trying to make our needs known when we can't speak the language, or know only a few words, can be both fun and frustrating, but certainly makes us think and function in new ways. Traveling to regions of great natural beauty, or of natural wonders, may be interesting but doesn't do much for us if we just go and ooh and aah. On the other hand, if we read or study about what we are seeing, it is much more worthwhile.

Collecting

Collecting is an activity that can generate excitement, while requiring learning and information about the items being accumulated. The amount of knowledge necessary depends on what is being collected and how it is obtained. Acquiring pretty sea shells by walking on the beach is different from evaluating a piece of outsider art and debating whether to buy it. Of course, if you decide to delve into sea shells and learn everything possible about the specimens you've found, it can be cognitively stimulating. And the pieces in a collection are often an impetus to learning. People can collect virtually anything, from bottle caps and typewriter ribbons, to Disney memorabilia and occupied Japan pottery, to Arts and Crafts furniture and contemporary art. For many kinds of collections, wealth is not a prerequisite, merely time and effort. To some people, the quest may be as important as owning a particular piece. There are newsletters and books about most collectible objects as well as organizations devoted to these objects.

Cognitive Training

As the value of cognitive stimulation to prevent dementia and cognitive decline in older people has been recognized, there have been some studies of formal programs that try to enhance brain function. These have occurred both in normal populations and patients with MCI and Alzheimer's disease, with the beneficial effects more pronounced in those who were cognitively intact.

One involved a sample of over 2,800 persons age 65 to 94 living independently within the community who were randomized into 4 groups of about 700 subjects each, 3 of which were given cognitive training interventions.[14] These consisted of 10 sessions, lasting 60 to 75 minutes, of group training over a 5 to 6 week period. Patients with cognitive impairment or severe medical problems were excluded. One group was given instructions designed to improve verbal episodic memory, another in reasoning ability to solve problems that follow a serial pattern and another in speed of processing with visual search and identification. The initial five sessions were devoted to strategy instruction, and individual and group exercises to practice the strategy. The last five sessions provided additional practice exercises. Eleven months after the training sessions, four booster sessions of 75 minutes each over a 2–3 week period were provided to 60 percent of the three trained groups selected randomly. There was a two year follow-up.

Each program generated an immediate effect in its corresponding cognitive domain and the vast majority of subjects remained independent regarding the tasks of daily living during the period of the study. Booster training further improved performance, particularly in terms of speed and reasoning. Though the impact of cognitive training did fall off over time, there was still a statistically significant effect over the full 2 years, with the trained individuals having better cognitive skills than the controls. Given the results of this study, the authors felt that cognitive training interventions have the potential to stabilize or improve expected age related cognitive decline that occurs in older people.

Cognitive-motor intervention (CMI) was also tried in small groups of patients with mild cognitive impairment, mild Alzheimer's disease and moderate Alzheimer's, who were taking cholinesterase inhibitors.[15] The patients were randomized with half of each group receiving psychosocial support plus cognitive-motor intervention and the other half psychomotor support alone. Cognitive-motor intervention entailed a structured program over a year of 103 sessions (twice weekly) of cognitive exercises with psychomotor and social activities. Evaluations were repeated at 1, 3, 6 and 12 months with a number of tests of cognitive ability, mood and functional activities. Those patients in the CMI group had maintained cognitive status at 6 months, with the control group declining significantly. At 12 months, though mood and behavior were maintained or improved, cognitive ability was not. This study showed that though CMI may be helpful in overall care of Alzheimer's patients, it does not have long-term efficacy in maintaining cognitive function.

Other plans for cognitive intervention in the normal elderly and patients with mild cognitive impairment are being utilized to try and bolster brain function, aid in the tasks of daily living and reduce the chances of dementia. Though there are proponents for some of these, for the most part they are expensive and labor intensive, and it may be difficult to disseminate these widely.

Though formal cognitive training may be valuable in preventing cognitive decline in individuals who have not yet entered the downward spiral of dementia, there are many activities we can engage in ourselves as we have detailed in this chapter. We must remember that if we continue to be intellectually stimulated, our brains will maintain their plasticity and ability to change, and we will keep increasing our synapses daily, delaying or preventing the loss of cognitive function.

Chapter 11

DIET AND SUBSTANCES THAT MAY REDUCE THE RISK OF DEMENTIA

Happy is the man that findeth wisdom
And the man that obtaineth understanding.

Proverbs 3:13

Eat, drink and be merry, for tomorrow we die.

A common saying

DIET

What we eat and drink affects how we live and die, and the status of our brains. In the fight against cognitive decline, the food we ingest daily is a major weapon. We have shown previously that vascular risk factors increase the chances of developing dementia independently of actual strokes or cerebrovascular disease which are also risk factors for dementia. Thus, anything in our diets that reduces cholesterol, athero-sclerosis, diabetes and hypertension aids in maintaining brain function. The so-called heart healthy diets that have been promulgated in books, magazines and on television to prevent coronary artery disease are also brain healthy diets.

Over the years, many different diets have been advocated to promote overall health and to specifically address vascular disease. With common sense, we can cull some ideas from these and come up with general rules regarding diet and dementia.

Remember that whole foods and fresh foods, which have not undergone changes and have no additives, are healthier than processed foods.

Stay away from bad fats. By that is meant avoiding saturated and trans fats as much as possible. These are most common in fried foods and baked goods, dairy products that have not reduced fat content and red meats. Ingesting large amounts of saturated fat or trans fats, and high total fats have been shown to heighten the risk of Alzheimer's disease. In laboratory animals, ingestion of saturated fats was found to increase the deposition of amyloid in the brain.[1] On the other hand, unsaturated, unhydrogenated fats are protective. The best of these may be monounsaturated fat found in olive oil, a staple of the so-called Mediterranean diet renowned for promoting longevity and clean arteries. Substituting olive oil for butter wherever acceptable is a smart objective, along with limiting fried foods and red meats.

Fish that are high in polyunsaturated fatty acids (PUFA) are of particular value as they decrease blood pressure, cholesterol and triglyceride levels, and significantly lower the risk of heart attacks and atherosclerosis. They also appear to protect against strokes and dementia. Both long chain n-3 PUFA and omega-3 PUFA such as docosahexaenoic acid (DHA) which are found in fish have this effect. DHA can also be manufactured within the body from its precursor n-3 PUFA. These compounds are essential components of the phospholipids in the neuronal membranes, and DHA is found in high levels in the parts of the brain and brain cells that are most metabolically active. They also appear to act as antioxidants and decrease inflammation. One prospective study conducted over 7 years in 815 community residents found that those who ate fish once per week or more had a 60 percent reduction in the risk of developing Alzheimer's disease compared to those who rarely or never ate fish.[2] A review article noted, "A high fish consumption tended to be inversely associated with cognitive impairment and decline."[3] In other words, the more fish consumed, the lower the chances of dementia. Another study, however, did not find any relationship between ingestion of various types of fats and the subsequent risk of developing dementia.[4]

Intake of fruits and vegetables also plays an important role in protecting the brain, and the more that is eaten, the better. Current recommendations are for people to have five or more portions of fruits and vegetables daily, or fruit juices. These are excellent sources of vitamins and various antioxidants such as flavonoids and polyphenols. Dark fruits and vegetables appear to be particularly rich in protective compounds. Thus, one should be eating different kinds of berries (blueberries, strawberries, raspberries, cranberries, blackberries) frequently, or drinking juices derived from berries. Grapes and grape juice or red wine are also good sources, as are cherries, plums and tomatoes. Apple juice concentrate appears to be rich in antioxidants as well, and able to prevent oxidative damage and decline in cognitive performance in transgenic mice according to a recent report.[5] But its efficacy in human subjects needs further evaluation. One large study that over 6.3 years followed 1,800 people who were free of dementia at baseline found that fruit and vegetable juices appeared to delay the onset of Alzheimer's disease in their population.[6] Green leafy vegetables are also essential as they provide B vitamins and folic acid as well as antioxidants, all of which help to sustain brain function.

Green and black tea are also excellent sources of antioxidants with both containing high levels of polyphenols and flavonoids. Green tea's active compounds are catechins, particularly epigallocatechin-3-gallate (EGCG), while black tea's are theaflavins and thea rubigens. They are all powerful antioxidants, effective at neutralizing free radicals and reducing oxidative stress, and may also increase insulin sensitivity and effectiveness. There is some suggestion that green and black tea may have neuroprotective properties over and above their actions as antioxidants. A recent study has also shown decreased amyloid production in transgenic Alzheimer's mice given EGCG, raising the possibility that a dietary supplement of this compound or green tea itself may be useful in the prophylaxis or treatment of Alzheimer's disease.[7] While regular intake of green or black tea may be helpful in delaying or preventing Alzheimer's, more data is necessary to confirm this.

Other elements of our diets also influence general health, atherosclerosis and cognitive function, but are not quite as important as the fat content and types of fat we ingest, and the amounts of fruits, vegetables and juices. Among these, whole grains, such as whole wheat or oatmeal and brown rice, are healthier for us than grains that have been processed, such as white breads and white rice, with their vitamins and minerals mostly removed. Having nuts as part of our diets is also worthwhile. Though high in calories, nuts are also high in monounsaturated and polyunsaturated fatty acids, the good kind of fats, and are a source of vitamins, minerals and antioxidants. Almonds, walnuts and pecans appear to be the best, but because they are rich in calories, total intake should be restricted. The amount of salt in our diets should also be limited, since it raises blood pressure in those predisposed and has no nutritional value. As mentioned previously, one or two drinks of an alcoholic beverage daily lowers the risk of dementia, while imbibing more may heighten the risk. Coffee consumption should also be reduced, as larger amounts are pro-inflammatory.

There should be minimal intake of foods containing simple carbohydrates because they increase insulin resistance and promote diabetes, making dementia more likely. Soda, candy, other sweets and processed foods containing refined sugar should be reduced. On the other hand, complex carbohydrates (dietary fibers and starches) found in grains, breads, cereals, pasta, brown rice and legumes (peas and beans) should be utilized for the major part of our caloric intake. Carbohydrates are burned by our cells to provide energy for metabolic processes and we could not survive without adequate amounts. (The surplus is stored in the liver or muscles to be used at a later time.) But the form of the carbohydrates we ingest is important when considering the possibility of developing diabetes or dementia.

Many of the above suggestions for food intake protective against dementia and cognitive decline fit into the Mediterranean diet that combats atherosclerosis and heart disease. In analyzing our own diets, we should focus on those foods and compounds that increase the risk of dementia, and those deficiencies that also increase the risk. Although we should try to consume adequate amounts of fish, vegetables, fruits, antioxidants, n-3 PUFA and the B vitamins in our diets, we should also be wary of a high caloric intake, high fat content, saturated fats and sweets.

SUBSTANCES THAT MAY REDUCE THE RISK OF DEMENTIA

Aspirin

Because of its action as an antiplatelet agent, causing diminished aggregation and clumping of platelets, and preventing clots (thrombi) from forming within the blood vessels, aspirin has been used for vascular prophylaxis for decades, to lower the risk of heart attacks and strokes. By decreasing strokes and cerebrovascular disease, and increasing blood flow and oxygenation to the brain, aspirin can reduce the incidence of cognitive decline and dementia as well. Though it also has significant anti-inflammatory effects and could work in the brain against amyloid, these would not appear to be the main ways it fights dementia. Unless there are specific contraindications, such as ulcers or aspirin sensitivity, I recommend that everyone over 50 take a baby aspirin (81 mg) daily, as the risk-reward ratio favors this approach. Aspirin is one of the major weapons in our arsenal in the battle against strokes and dementia.

Non-Steroidals (NSAIDs)

A chronic inflammatory response to beta-amyloid in the brains of Alzheimer's patients is part of the pathologic process, and it is believed that some of the neuronal damage occurs because of this. In addition, elevated serum markers of inflammation, such as C-reactive protein (CRP) and interleukin 6, have been shown to be associated with cognitive decline in well functioning elderly people. These findings led investigators to wonder if the use of anti-inflammatory drugs would provide protection against dementia. A number of population-based studies demonstrated that people who took non-steroidals regularly appeared to have a lowered incidence of dementia.[8] Another study followed close to 7,000 cognitively normal older individuals for an average of 6.8 years.[9] Only 1.3 percent of those who used NSAIDs for more than 24 months developed dementia, compared to 8.2 percent of those who did not. A different report suggested that only the long-term use of NSAIDs before the onset of cognitive decline would provide protection from dementia.[10] The data in a number of other studies was somewhat contradictory, but still favoring a protective effect of NSAIDs.

To try and settle the question, the ADAPT study (Alzheimer's Disease Anti-inflammatory Prevention Trail) with naproxen and Celebrex (celecoxib) was undertaken at multiple centers. Unfortunately, this had to be stopped because of an apparent linkage of these medications to cardiovascular events.[11] At present the jury is out in terms of whether NSAIDs really are protective against dementia (and if they are, when, how long and how much should be taken) and whether the potential benefits outweigh possible adverse occurrences. These include heartburn, possible ulcers and GI bleeding, and rarely kidney or liver damage. If a person is at high risk of developing Alzheimer's disease, it may be worthwhile taking ibuprofen for prophylaxis, 400–600 mg daily, with awareness of the possible complications that can occur.

As mentioned in Chapter 3, an NSAID analogue, flurizan (R-flurbiprofen) is currently undergoing clinical testing in patients with Alzheimer's disease after appearing effective in transgenic mice. In addition to reducing inflammation, it also appears to lower levels of beta-amyloid 42, possibly by affecting its production through gamma secretase pathways. Other NSAIDs may work in a similar fashion and in the future newer variants may be tried as well.

Of interest, another study has suggested that ibuprofen may be protective against Parkinson's disease.[12] Patients (147,000) participating in an American Cancer Society prevention study were shown to have a 38 percent reduced risk of developing Parkinson's if they took ibuprofen daily during the previous year, compared to nonusers. There was a 35 percent reduction if they took two or more pills weekly. The same effect, however, was not found for other NSAIDs. Further work needs to be done to verify this data.

Ginko Biloba

Ginko biloba is a substance derived from the leaf of a tropical plant of the same name, marketed over-the-counter in the United States as a dietary supplement. For decades it has been widely used, mainly by older people because of a popular belief that it improved cognitive function, particularly memory, and prevented Alzheimer's disease. It contains flavonoids and terpenoids which have antioxidant properties and neutralize free radicals. In addition, there have been claims that ginko acts as a neuroprotective agent—heightens metabolism efficiency, is a membrane stabilizer, relaxes the endothelium of the arteries, increases cerebral blood flow and oxygen uptake, elevates choline levels in the hippocampus, regulates neurotransmitters and possibly inhibits beta-amyloid deposition.[13] Another action is the reduction of platelet adhesion or stickiness—similar to aspirin—reducing clotting and promoting easier blood flow. Because of this effect, bleeding may occur if it is used in patients who are already taking other agents that lessen platelet adhesion, or anticoagulants. But generally, its is considered a safe substance for most people, with occasional diarrhea, nausea and headache.

Besides its utilization to prevent and treat Alzheimer's, ginko is employed for vascular dementia and peripheral arterial disease. Past studies have suggested some modest efficacy in modulating the symptoms of dementia and cerebrovascular insufficiency, particularly in mild to moderate Alzheimer's disease. But three trials using more stringent modern criteria were inconclusive regarding benefits in age-related memory problems and Alzheimer's, though in higher doses it may have improved memory in a normal population. Larger randomized, controlled studies are needed to finally decide its worth and a number of these trials are now going on. Currently, however, its value both for prophylaxis and treatment of memory problems and dementia is unclear.

Selegiline (Deprenyl)

Selegiline is a selective MAO-B inhibitor that has been used for some time in the treatment of Parkinson's disease. In this condition, it works as a neuroprotective substance and also appears to increase the neurotransmitter dopamine which is deficient. It is thought by some investigators that it may offer protection in mild cognitive impairment against the development of Alzheimer's, and delay progression when Alzheimer's is present. Whether it will prevent the onset of dementia in cognitively normal older people is uncertain, though claims have been made to that effect. It is believed by some that it may improve cognitive performance in healthy normals.

Selegiline reduces oxidative stress and DNA damage by decreasing the production of hydrogen peroxide and free radicals, partially by stimulating the release of the enzyme superoxide dismutase (SOD). It is also felt that it protects against excitotoxic damage from the neurotransmitter glutamate. The mitochondria, which are the minute factories within the cells where many metabolic processes occur, are preserved by selegiline due to its effects on mitochondrial membrane permeability. Hippocampal neurons, which play a major role in short-term memory, may be protected by selegiline, and it results in an elevation of BDNF (brain derived neurotrophic factor) and other growth factors which are neuroprotective. An allied compound which is being used experimentally in Parkinson's works in a similar fashion. Besides possibly enhancing memory and learning, selegiline may also act as an antidepressant and affect mood. Side effects from this compound are relatively mild when they occur, and include dizziness, dry mouth and various GI symptoms. Selegiline is a prescription medication and can only be utilized under a physician's supervision. Although it appears to have some beneficial effects, there is not enough hard evidence yet to warrant its routine use in the general population to delay or prevent dementia.

Statin Drugs—3-HMG Coenzyme A Reductase Inhibitors (Lipitor, Mevacor, Zocor, Pravachol, Crestor, etc.)

Though the final conclusion about the value of statin drugs in protecting against dementia remains open, these compounds could potentially work in a number of ways. As noted in Chapter 3, statin use appears to diminish the incidence of strokes by several mechanisms. Just on that basis alone, one would expect a decreased risk of dementia in people taking statins. But it is also believed that statins may modulate Alzheimer's pathology directly by inhibiting beta amyloid production and by changing amyloid precursor protein pathways. The statins' anti-inflammatory and antioxidative effects may also impact the Alzheimer's process, and they are believed by some to be neuroprotective.[14]

One large study involving over 9,000 patients found that another type of lipid lowering agent besides statins (fibrate) was also effective in lowering the prevalence of dementia.[15] Another report observed that statin use did not influence cognitive function over a period of 6 to 8 years, with no significant difference in mini-mental states in the treated group of 290 patients and the control group.[16]

There have also been some reports of statin use causing impairment of memory and cognitive function in a small percentage of people taking these drugs.[17] This is apparently an infrequent occurrence and is usually reversible when the drug is discontinued. Cognitive disturbances are more common and more profound in the elderly, in whom the overall benefits of statins and lowering cholesterol are not as clear cut. At this time, the evidence on the use of statins to prevent dementia remains inconclusive. However, because they reduce cholesterol and appear to diminish the incidence of strokes, it would seem to be worthwhile treating anyone at risk for dementia who has an elevated or even borderline cholesterol with these drugs. Whether they will be found in the future to play a direct role in reducing the amyloid burden in Alzheimer's patients remains to be seen.

Vitamins E and C

The data on the effectiveness of vitamin E in preventing cognitive decline and dementia is also controversial. Although for years there was excitement about the presumed benefits of vitamin E in neurodegenerative diseases, recent data has not been supportive. Vitamin E is an antioxidant and is felt to limit free radical formation and oxidative stress in the brain, and from a theoretical standpoint, could be neuroprotective. It was shown in one trial of patients with Alzheimer's published in 1997 to slow progression of the disease.[18] In another study of nearly 3,000 older community residents over a seven year period, the rate of cognitive decline was reduced 36 percent in the quartile with the highest vitamin E intake versus the lowest quartile.[19] This was true both for foods containing vitamin E and supplements. Another large community study found a trend toward reduced Alzheimer's disease in people taking vitamin E supplements, or vitamin E in combination with vitamin C.[20] Because of these and other studies, and because it is inexpensive and was believed to be relatively safe, it was widely used both in patients with Alzheimer's and in normal people for primary prevention.[21] However, in a trial of 769 subjects with the amnestic form of mild cognitive impairment treated with 2,000 units of vitamin E or donepizil, progression to Alzheimer's disease was no different in the group taking vitamin E compared to the placebo group.[22]

There is also some evidence that vitamin E may provide protection from the neuronal degeneration seen in Parkinson's disease by reducing oxidative stress. Though it has been utilized for treatment, and in asymptomatic subjects to potentially lower the risk of developing this condition, the data about its benefits has been inconsistent. In a large prospective study utilizing food frequency questionnaires, where over 76,000 women and over 47,000 men were followed for 14 years and 12 years respectively, total vitamin E intake and the use of vitamin E supplements did not affect the development of Parkinson's disease.[23] However, high dietary intake of vitamin E from foods rich in this substance and consumption of nuts did appear to reduce the risk of Parkinson's.

Vitamin E has been known to prolong clotting times and in rare cases can cause abnormal bleeding. Reports have suggested a possible increase in all-cause mortality as well as coronary events in people who take high doses of vitamin E. With the value of vitamin E in the prevention of cognitive decline and dementia open to question, and its safety in high doses remaining an issue, the question of where and when it should be employed has not been settled. Smaller doses of vitamin E (200–400 IU) daily are probably okay to use, though it is uncertain how much protection this will provide. Vitamin C is not as strong an antioxidant as vitamin E, but there has been some suggestion that the two work together, and that vitamin E's effects are potentiated by C.

Another recent large prospective study suggests that in order to be truly effective in reducing the risk of Alzheimer's, vitamin E has to be obtained from natural sources rather than supplements.[24] The latter contains mainly alpha tocopherol, while food has four different forms of tocopherol. The protective effect of vitamin E may be related to intake of the combined forms which may act synergistically, increasing generation of antioxidant proteins such as superoxide dismutase. Gamma tocopherol, which has very potent anti-inflammatory properties and is a major free radical scavenger, is generally not found in pills. The most important food sources for vitamin E are vegetable and seed oils, with alpha tocopherol most abundant in sunflower and wheat germ oils, and gamma tocopherol found most in corn and soybean oils. In this study, it was shown that vitamin E intake from food was linearly and inversely associated with Alzheimer's incidence; in other words, the greater the intake, the less the chances of developing the disease. Though more testing of this hypothesis is necessary, it may be that we're simply not getting our vitamin E from the right sources.

Vitamin B12, Vitamin B6 and Folic Acid (folate)

Elevated homocysteine levels in the blood are linked to an increased risk of coronary artery disease and strokes. In over 1,000 normal elderly subjects who were part of the Framingham study, a correlation was also found between high homocysteine levels and both dementia in general and Alzheimer's in particular.[25] This would appear to be a modifiable risk factor for dementia since homocysteine levels can be reduced by using folic acid. However, another report suggested that elevated homocysteine in Alzheimer's patients might be related to vascular disease rather than the Alzheimer's pathology.[26] (Of course, we already know that cerebrovascular disease and strokes can result in an unmasking of Alzheimer's symptoms.) These investigators also found that vitamin B6 levels were reduced in patients with Alzheimer's. An analysis hypothesized that homocysteine could have a primary effect on the microcirculation of the brain or could be toxic to brain cells.[27] A different study observed that subjects with low levels of either B12 or folate were twice as likely as normals to acquire Alzheimer's disease.[28]

For many years it has been known that patients with very low B12 levels can develop dementia along with degeneration of tracts in the spinal cord and peripheral nerve damage. Though rare at present, this constellation was seen in the past in patients with pernicious anemia who had difficulty absorbing vitamin B12, and was called combined system disease. Because of its effect in reducing homocysteine, folic acid or folate also appears to influence the possibility of developing dementia, as do low levels of vitamin B6. However, there was one report suggesting that folic acid supplements at or above 400 micrograms, or a diet high in folate, might be risk factors for cognitive decline. At present, overall evidence is equivocal about the benefit of folate and it is uncertain whether taking B6, B12 and folic acid to reduce the risk of dementia. There are small quantities of these three substances in multivitamin pills. It is not known whether additional supplementation may be of value. However, there are pills available that combine these three vitamins in higher doses than the usual multivitamin (folic acid 0.4–1 mg, vitamin B6 25–100 mg, vitamin B12 500–1000mcg).

Vitamin B3 (Niacin)

Low dietary intake of niacin has been shown in some studies to be correlated with cognitive decline and Alzheimer's disease.[29] A severe deficiency causes pellagra with diarrhea, dermatitis, dementia and a swollen red tongue, seen in developing countries as part of the spectrum of malnutrition. In the Western world, it is usually associated with alcoholism. B3, like all the B vitamins, is water soluble and a potent antioxidant linked to the production of cellular energy, metabolism of fats and proteins and elimination of toxins. It is also involved in DNA synthesis and repair, neural cell signaling, improves circulation and helps to reduce cholesterol levels.

Several studies have shown that the risk of cognitive decline and dementia appears lowest in those subjects with the highest daily consumption of niacin. This suggests that increasing niacin intake may offer some protection against the development of Alzheimer's and dementia. However, large doses of niacin can cause liver damage, ulcers, skin rashes, flushing and dizziness, so one should be cautious. Though 1,000 mg daily or even more may be used to reduce serum cholesterol, 100 to 300 mg is probably more reasonable for its effects on the brain.

Coenzyme Q10 (Ubiquinone)

Coenzyme Q10 is a vitamin-like compound that is fat soluble and plays a role in the generation of energy within the mitochondria of the cell. It is contained in a number of foods such as beef, organ meats, soy oil, peanuts and sardines, but is also synthesized by the body. No significant side effects or toxicity have been associated with it. It has antioxidant properties, attacking free radicals and protecting against oxidative stress. Levels of Q10 are reduced with aging, and statin usage may block its synthesis and reduce levels as well. Heart failure may be helped by Q10. The dosages that people have used vary from 10 to 50 mg three times daily, to double or triple the higher amount.

The value of Coenzyme Q10 in neurodegenerative diseases is unclear. There have been reports of its slowing the progression of Parkinson's disease,[30] and of possibly slowing the decline in Huntington's.[31] Low levels of Q10 have been found in Lewy body disease, suggesting this may play a role in its development. But that needs further study. Questions have also been raised about its benefits in Alzheimer's disease. However, one study did not find any difference in the levels of Coenzyme Q10 in patients with Alzheimer's or vascular dementia compared to controls.[32] At this time, though we do not have hard evidence of Coenzyme Q10 being helpful in treating any form of dementia, or in preventing its occurrence, the possibility remains open.

Turmeric (Curcumin)

Curcumin is a polyphenolic ingredient of curry powder derived from the plant curcuma longa and is not related to the spice cumin. With potent antioxidant and anti-inflammatory properties, curcumin structurally resembles amyloid binding dyes, is a free radical scavenger and suppresses oxidative damage, inflammation and amyloid accumulation. It also lowers cholesterol and raises HDL cholesterol. In both cell cultures and mice studies, it has been shown to block beta-amyloid aggregation and fibril formation,[33] and previously formed fibrils appear to be broken up by it. Indeed, curcumin appears to play a role in many pathways within the neuron related to amyloid and is protective of the cell. In India where it is widely used as an ingredient of curry, there appears to be a lower incidence of Alzheimer's in the elderly population. Though curcumin looks quite promising, at this time the proper dosage and potential side effects have not been defined, though it seems to have a favorable toxicity profile. A small clinical trial is now underway sponsored by the NIH to test safety and efficacy of two standard doses of curcumin in mild to moderate Alzheimer's patients. If it is found to be safe, it may be a substance that can be used to treat Alzheimer's disease and possibly other dementias. It may also be a preventative for those who are at high risk for Alzheimer's, or even for the general population from midlife on as a possible way to stabilize cognitive function.

Alcohol

As previously mentioned, excessive alcohol damages neurons and accelerates cognitive decline. However, moderate alcohol intake appears to be protective of intellectual abilities as shown in the Nurse's Health Study where over 11,000 women had cognition evaluated over 2 years.[34] (Moderate was defined as about one drink daily—15 gms or half an ounce.) There was no difference in the type of alcohol ingested. Other studies have confirmed this effect in both men and women, though some have suggested that wine specifically is beneficial.[35] The reason for alcohol's effect is unclear with one hypothesis citing its known ability to reduce vascular disease. Alcohol appears to increase blood levels of HDL cholesterol, the so-called good cholesterol, and diminishes blood clotting agents such as fibrinogen. Because of this, it offers some protection against heart attacks and may also protect against the small subclinical strokes that cumulatively damage the brain. Thus the incidence of both Alzheimer's and vascular dementia may be reduced. The key here is moderate intake.

ACE Inhibitors

ACE (angiotensin converting enzyme) inhibitors are a class of drugs used to treat high blood pressure. According to one study, brain penetrating ACE inhibitors (captopril and perindopril) appeared to decrease the incidence of Alzheimer's in elderly hypertensive patients.[36] The question is whether this was due to lowering of the blood pressure and vascular risk factors, or because of some direct effect on the disease process itself. There is evidence that components of the renin-angiotensin system may be important in learning and memory, and angiotensin converting enzyme is apparently found in higher amounts than expected in the hippocampus and frontal cortex of patients with Alzheimer's. It has also been shown that ACE inhibitors may slow cognitive decline in patients with Alzheimer's and hypertension, independent of a reduction in blood pressure. This suggests there may be enhancement of the renin-angiotensin system within the brain by ACE inhibitors. There is not enough confirmatory data yet to have all Alzheimer's patients take brain penetrating ACE inhibitors, but if they do have hypertension, this would certainly be the preferred mode of treatment. Similarly, hypertensive patients who have mild cognitive impairment, or are at risk for developing dementia, should be using these compounds.

Testosterone

As men age, their production of testosterone gradually declines. Some recent studies have suggested that low levels of testosterone in older men are associated with a greater risk of Alzheimer's disease.[37] Male hormones, also known as androgens, may influence brain function directly through their effect on androgen receptors in the brain, or may be converted to estradiol, the female sex hormone, and interact with the estrogen receptors.[38] In laboratory animals, testosterone has been shown to decrease the formation of beta-amyloid and the pathologic changes in tau protein, both of which are important elements in Alzheimer's. Testosterone supplements have also been found to improve memory and cognitive function in healthy older men.[39] Though there are some other positive physiologic effects for men who take testosterone when they are older, such as improved strength, muscle mass, stamina and sex drive, there are also some potential negative sequelae, among which are joint pains, liver problems and an increase in prostate cancer. At this time, the information available does not warrant taking testosterone to prevent or treat Alzheimer's, or dementia in general.

Estrogen

There was a time in the not so distant past when hormone replacement therapy in women, in addition to treating menopausal symptoms, was perceived as a panacea for aging, with all its associated diseases and disorders. Unfortunately, the common wisdom has been proven wrong. Rather than reducing the incidence of heart attacks, strokes and dementia among other problems, hormone replacement increases the risks and is potentially harmful. In the Women's Health Initiative Memory Study which was published in 2003 and 2004, and involved over 4,500 cognitively intact women, the use of estrogen to protect against dementia was put to bed.[40] Not only did hormone replacement not offer protection, but it was shown also to heighten the possibility of older women developing dementia. The risk was increased for dementia overall and the various subgroups. It also did not protect against mild cognitive impairment. And the outcome was the same whether estrogen was used alone or combined with progestin. Although hormone replacement therapy may be helpful for alleviating the symptoms of menopause, there are certainly long-term risks to be considered.

Silica

There have been reports of high levels of silica (component of sand) in drinking water reducing the risk of intellectual decline.[41] Over 7,500 older women in France had cognitive evaluations correlated with the composition of the water they drank. The subjects who scored highest had higher amounts of silica in their water. In addition, in a follow-up of up to 7 years, women who developed Alzheimer's were found to have a low intake of silica. Though the mechanism of action for the presumed protection silica offers is unknown, it was hypothesized that this was related to aluminum in some way. This needs further study before silica intake can be suggested as a way to reduce dementia.

DHA (Docosahexanoic Acid)

Omega 3 fatty acids and DHA were discussed earlier in this chapter in terms of dietary intake and their protective effect against dementia. Studies thus far favor a role for them in reducing the risk of dementia in general and Alzheimer's specifically. Though ingesting the natural foods that contain these substances would be the best way to get them, there are now DHA enriched foods and eggs fortified with DHA available, as well as fish oil capsules. The old-fashioned liquid cod liver oil is also an excellent source of omega 3 fatty acids and DHA (900 mg/teaspoon), showing us that perhaps our mothers knew what they were talking about. However, there is not yet enough data to recommend supplementation of DHA and omega 3s to protect against dementia nor what the appropriate doses should be. There are ongoing studies, however, that should resolve these questions.

Antioxidants

In every neurodegenerative disorder, free radicals are felt to be critical players, damaging and destroying neurons. Compounds that have antioxidant properties are considered to be of particular importance in preventing Alzheimer's, Parkinson's and other dementias because of their effect on free radicals and the reduction of oxidative stress which make them neuroprotective. We have mentioned many of them individually and as components of foods, including vitamin E, vitamin C, niacin, DHA and Omega 3 fatty acids, turmeric, Coenzyme Q10, biofavonoids, polyphenols and so forth. There are many other substances with these properties, such as vitamin D, carotinoids, acetyl l-carnitine and so forth, that we have not discussed. Supplements are available for many of these, but the benefits have usually not been well defined, except for the knowledge that they are antioxidants. There have been some suggestions that antioxidant cocktails containing multiple compounds may be the best way to protect against dementia and the other diseases of aging, but the evidence for this has not been forthcoming. Listed below are some other antioxidants.

Grape seed extract is a natural plant substance containing bioflavonoids and polyphenols. Its activity is mostly mediated through oligomeric proanthocyanidans (procyanidolic oligomers) which are more powerful antioxidants than vitamins E and C. Grape seed extract may interact with anticoagulants and cholesterol lowering drugs, so caution is advised if these medications are being utilized. The effective dose is really unknown, but the companies that make these supplements suggest 50–200 mg daily, with older individuals requiring the highest amounts. Further evaluation is necessary to see if the presumed benefits are valid.

Resveratrol is another naturally occurring antioxidant found in red wine and peanuts that is available in supplements. It is felt to be of possible value in combating atherosclerosis and may offer some protection against dementia. The current information, however, does not support regular usage.

Alpha lipoic acid (ALA) is yet another compound with antioxidant properties that has gained popularity as an alternative method for the prevention and treatment of Alzheimer's and other neurodegenerative diseases, as well as diabetes, heart disease and strokes. ALA is important in protecting mitochondrial function and genetic material in the cells. It is a strong antioxidant that appears to attack a wide variety of free radicals in different organ systems including the brain. After being given a substance that produces an Alzheimer's type dementia, mice treated with ALA or trans resveratrol were found to have improved memory function compared to controls.[42] Little free ALA is available in our bodies, unless supplements are utilized. There is still not enough evidence to advise taking it, and the optimum dosage is uncertain, though 100–600 mg per day are being suggested by manufacturers.

Value has also been claimed for garlic extract and cinnamon which do have antioxidant properties in fighting dementia, but evidence for this is lacking.

The body constantly produces and utilizes its own antioxidants in the fight against free radicals and oxidative stress. As we age, we are attacked by more free radicals and the oxidative stress increases. At the same time, our tissues may be manufacturing less antioxidants than previously. While all of the antioxidants that are ingested have theoretical value, the question is whether these compounds reach high enough concentrations in the target organs, such as the brain, to have a significant effect on those cells that are stressed and affect the disease processes. Scientific studies continue and we are still learning.

In summary, protection against dementia and cognitive decline may be forthcoming by eating fish and consuming a diet rich in fruits and vegetables. Saturated fats, trans fats and simple carbohydrates are to be avoided. Olive oil, whole grains and nuts, along with green and black tea are beneficial. The usefulness of the various vitamins, food supplements and other substances has been described above.

Possibly in the future, after more studies have been performed and more information is available, we may find that in addition to exercise and cognitive stimulation, several pills taken each morning with breakfast may provide us with neuroprotection and eliminate dementia the way rheumatic fever was erased with penicillin.

AFTERWORD

To understand others is to be knowledgeable
To understand yourself is to be wise.

Te Tao Ching[1]

There are no second acts in American lives.

F. Scott Fitzgerald

Like being enveloped by an approaching fog, cognitive decline and dementia are potential problems for all of us as we grow older, with increasing likelihood of our minds being affected with every year that passes. But as we have demonstrated in this book, there are ways for us to dissipate this fog or prevent it from forming. We do have considerable control over our minds and bodies, and can influence the processes that result in dementia if we take the appropriate steps. Though it is better if we initiate a program of exercise, cognitive stimulation and proper diet early, it is never too late to start, for unless the curtain of dementia has already descended, we will derive benefits.

The key word for us is discipline, for activities are required on a daily basis that entail time and effort, with the desired effects perhaps not evident for decades. Still, it is important that we commit ourselves to the necessary tasks, for if we keep procrastinating, it may be too late, and we may never reap the benefits we desire.

If you are already moving forward on that long road, do not stop. If you haven't yet begun your trek, start now. As the old Chinese proverb notes, "a journey of a thousand miles begins with a single step." The journey should continue until we die.

NOTES

PREFACE

1. *The Penguin Book of Japanese Verse*, Translated by Geoffrey Bownas and Anthony Thwaite, New York, 1983, p. 80.

CHAPTER 1: INTRODUCTION

1. S. Burner et al., "Nation's health care expenditures projections through 2030," *Health Care Financing Review*, 1992, 14, 1: 4.

2. Paul Solomon and Andrew Budson, "Alzheimer's disease," *Clinical Symposia*, 2003, 54, 1: 5.

3. Robert Nussbaum and Christopher Ellis, "Alzheimer's disease and Parkinson's disease," *N Engl J Med*, 2003, 348: 1356–1364.

4. G. Ravaglia et al., "Incidence and etiology of dementia in a large elderly Italian population," *Neurology*, 2005, 64: 1525–1530.

5. A. Lobo et al., "Prevalence of dementia and major subtypes in Europe. A collaborative study of population-based cohorts," *Neurology*, 2000, 54(Suppl 5): S4–9.

6. Andrew Budson and Bruce Price, "Memory Dysfunction," *N Engl J Med*, 2005, 353: 696–699.

7. Niels Prins et al., "Cerebral white matter lesions and the risk of dementia," *Arch Neurol*, 2004, 61: 1531–1534; S. Vermeer et al., "Silent brain infarcts and the risk of dementia and cognitive decline," *N Engl J Med*, 2003, 348: 1215–1222; Gustavo Roman "Age-associated white matter lesions and dementia," *Arch Neurol*, 2004, 61: 1503–1504.

8. R.A. Whitmer et al., "Midlife cardiovascular risk factors and risk of dementia in late life," *Neurology*, 2005, 64: 277–281.

9. Zoe Arvanitakis et al., "Diabetes mellitus and risk of Alzheimer disease and decline in cognitive function," *Arch Neurol*, 2004, 61: 661–666.

10. C. Justin Romano, "Obesity—A modifiable risk factor for Alzheimer's disease," *Neurology Reviews*, September 2004: 30.

11. Sudha Seshadri et al., "Plasma homocysteine as a risk factor for dementia and Alzheimer's disease," *N Engl J Med*, 2002, 346: 476–483; Marianne Engelhart et al., "Inflammatory proteins in plasma and the risk of dementia," *Arch Neuro*, 2004, 61: 668–672.

12. C. Dufouil et al., "APOE genotype, cholesterol level, lipid-lowering treatment, and dementia," *Neurology*, 2005, 64: 1531–1538; Christiane Reitz et al., "Relation of plasma lipids to Alzheimer's disease and vascular dementia," *Arch Neurol*, 2004, 61: 705–714.

13. C. Blair et al., "APOE gentype and cognitive decline in a middle aged cohort," *Neurology*, 2005, 64: 268–276.

14. A. Sundstrom et al., "APOE influences on neuropsychological function after mild head injury," *Neurology*, 2004, 62: 1963–1966; R. Caselli et al., "Longitudinal changes in cognition and behavior in asymptomatic carriers of the APOE e4 allele," *Neurology*, 2004, 62: 1990–1995.

15. Zaldy Sy Tan et al., "Bone mineral density and the risk of Alzheimer's disease," *Arch Neurol*, 2005, 62: 107–111.

16. ADM van Osch Liesbeth et al., "Low thyroid-stimulating hormone as an independent risk factor for Alzheimer's disease," *Neurology*, 2004, 62: 1967–1971.

17. R. Stewart et al., "A 32-year prospective study of change in body weight and incident dementia," *Arch Neurol*, 2005, 62: 55–60; Michael Grundman, "Weight loss in the elderly may be a sign of impending dementia," *Arch Neurol*, 2005, 62: 20–22.

18. M.F. Folstein, S.E. Folstein, P.R. McHugh, " 'Mini-Mental State': A practical method for grading cognitive states of patients for the clinician," *J Psychiatr Res*, 1975, 12: 189–198.

19. Mark Bondi et al., "FMRI evidence of compensatory mechanisms in older adults at genetic risk of Alzheimer's disease," *Neurology*, 2005, 64: 501–508.

20. Bruce Reed et al., "Effects of white matter lesions and lacunes on cortical function," *Arch Neurol*, 2004, 61: 1545–1550.

CHAPTER 2: CONFOUNDERS OF DEMENTIA: NORMAL AGING, MILD COGNITIVE IMPAIRMENT AND PSEUDO-DEMENTIA

1. May Sarton, *Kinds of Love*, W.W. Norton & Company, New York, 1994, p. 186.

2. David Drachman, "Do we have brain to spare?," *Neurology*, 2005, 64: 2004–2005.

3. Debra Hughes, "Accelerating factors in age-related atrophy," *Neurology Reviews*, September, 2004: 9.

4. C. Enzinger et al., "Risk factors for progression of brain atrophy in aging," *Neurology*, 2005, 64: 1704–1711.

5. Paul Coleman et al., "A focus on the synapse for neuroprotection in Alzheimer disease and other dementias," *Neurology*, 2004, 63: 1155–1162.

6. Leonard Hayflick, *How and Why We Age*, Ballantine Books, New York, 1996, p. 165.

7. Claudia Kawas, "Early Alzheimer's disease," *N Engl J Med*, 2003, 349: 1056–1063.

8. N.W. Milgram et al., "Learning ability in aged beagle dogs is preserved by behavioral enrichment and dietary fortification," *Neurobiology of Aging*, 2005, 26: 77–90; Nicholas Bakalar, "It can be done: Scientists teach old dogs new tricks," *New York Times* 2/6/05, Science Section, p. 1.

9. Larry Schuster, "Dementia experts debate diagnosis of mild cognitive impairment," *Neurology Today*, July 2004: p. 18.

10. C.A. Luis et al., "Mild cognitive impairment. Directions for future research," *Neurology*, 2003, 61: 438–444.

11. Masahiro Maruyama et al., "Cerebrospinal fluid tau protein and periventricular white matter lesions in patients with mild cognitive impairment," *Arch Neurol*, 2004, 61: 716–720.

12. Esther Korf et al., "Medial temporal lobe atrophy on MRI predicts dementia in patients with mild cognitive impairment," *Neurology*, 2004, 63: 94–100.

13. Schuster, "Dementia experts," *Neurology Today*. See note 9.

14. J. Olazaran et al., "Benefits of cognitive-motor intervention in MCI and mild to moderate Alzheimer's disease," *Neurology*, 2004, 63: 2348–2353.

15. R. Peterson, et al., "Mild cognitive impairment. Clinical characterization and outcome," *Arch Neurol*, 1999, 56: 303–308.

16. Martin Lehmann et al., "Vitamin B12-B6-folate treatment improves blood-brain barrier function in patients with hyperhomocysteinaemia and mild cognitive impairment," *Dement Geriatr Cogn Disord*, 2003, 16: 145–150.

17. Oliver Sacks and Melanie Shulman, "Steroid dementia: An overlooked diagnosis," *Neurology*, 2005, 64: 707–709.

18. O. Sedlaczek et al., "Detection of delayed focal MR changes in the lateral hippocampus in transient global amnesia," *Neurology*, 2004, 62: 2165–2170.

CHAPTER 3: ALZHEIMER'S DISEASE

1. Lao-Tzu, *Te Tao Ching*, Translated by Robert Hendricks, Ballantine Books, New York, 1989, p. 9.

2. Clauda Kawas, "Early Alzheimer's disease," *N Engl J Med*, 2003, 349: 1056–1063; Jeffrey Cummings, "Alzheimer's disease," *N Engl J Med*, 2004, 351: 56–67.

3. Dennis Selkoe, "Defining molecular targets to prevent Alzheimer's disease," *Arch Neurol*, 2005, 62: 192–195.

4. Ibid.

5. H. Houston Merritt, *A Textbook of Neurology*, 5th edition, 1973, Lea and Febeger, Philadelphia, p. 443.

6. Sir Francis Walshe, *Diseases of the Nervous System*, 9th edition, 1958, The Williams and Wilkins Company, Baltimore, MD; Lord Russell Brain, *Diseases of the Nervous System*, 6th edition, 1962, Oxford University Press, London.

7. Gunter Haase, *Diseases Presenting as Dementia. Contemporary Neurology Series*, F.A. Davis Company, Philadelphia, 1971, Chapter 10, p. 165.

8. Lan Xiong, Claudia Gaspar and Guy Rouleau, "Genetics of Alzheimer's disease and research frontiers in dementia," *Geriatrics Aging*, 2005, 8: 31–35.

9. "Researchers work toward development of Alzheimer's vaccine," *New York-Presbyterian Neurosciences*, Spring 2005: 4–5.

10. Dennis Selkoe, "Defining molecular targets to prevent Alzheimer's disease," *Arch Neurol*, 2005, 62: 192–195.

11. G.S. Watson et al., "Insulin increases CSF amyloid beta 42 levels in normal adults," *Neurology*, 2003, 60: 1988–1903.

12. Suzanne de la Monte, "Is Alzheimer's a Type 3 Diabetes?," *Alzheimer's Research Forum*, Live Discussion Transcript, April 14, 2005.

13. Mark A. Fishel et al., "Hyperinsulinemia provokes synchronous increases in central inflammation and beta-amyloid in normal adults," *Arch Neurol*, 2005, 62: 1539–1544.

14. P. Tiraboschi et al., "The importance of neuritic plaques and tangles to the development and evolution of AD," *Neurology*, 2004, 62: 1984–1989.

15. Paul Coleman et al., "A focus on the synapse for neuroprotection in Alzheimer disease and other dementias," *Neurology*, 2004, 63: 1155–1162.

16. Cummings, "Alzheimer's disease," *N Engl J Med*, 2004. See note 2.

17. Kurt Samson, "New technology tags biomarker for early Alzheimer's disease," *Neurology Today*, April 2005: 65–66.

18. Jeffrey Cummings, "Treatment of Alzheimer's disease: Current and future theropeutic approaches," *Reviews In Neurological Diseases*, 2004, Volume 1, 2: 60–69.

19. Michael Ehrenstein, Elizabeth Jury and Claudia Mauri, "Statins for atherosclerosis—As good as it gets?," *N Engl J Med* 2005, 352: 73–75; Paul Ridker et al., "C-Reactive protein levels and outcomes after statin therapy," *N Engl J Med*, 2005, 352: 20–28.

20. Benjamin Wolozin et al., "Decreased prevalence of Alzheimer disease associated with 3-hydroxy-3-methyglutaryl coenzyme a reductase inhibitors,"

Arch Neurol, 2000, 57: 1439–1443; G. Li et al., "Statin therapy and risk of dementia in the elderly," *Neurology*, 2004, 63: 1624–1628; D. Larry Sparks et al., "Atorvastatin for the treatment of mild to moderate Alzheimer disease," *Arch Neurol*, 2005, 62: 753–757.

21. Lawrence Honig, Walter Kukull and Richard Mayeux, "Atherosclerosis and AD," *Neurology*, 2005, 64: 494–500.

22. T. Ohrui et al., "Effects of brain-penetrating ACE inhibitors on Alzheimer's disease progression," *Neurology*, 2004, 63: 1324–1325.

23. A. Ueki, "The Japanese diet trial for patients with Alzheimer's disease," Presentation at the Boston Alzheimer's Symposium, October 21, 2005.

24. Sangram Sisodia, "Molecular neurobiology of AD," Grand Rounds, Harvard Medical School, October 20, 2005.

25. Karlene Ball et al., "Effects of cognitive training interventions with older adults," *JAMA*, 2002, 288: 2271–2281.

26. Kawas, "Early Alzheimer's disease," *N Engl J Med*; Cummings, "Alzheimer's disease," *N Engl J Med*. See note 2.

27. Michelle Sullivan, "U.K. eyes limits for dementia drugs," *Clincal Neurology News*, April 2005: 1–10.

28. H. Feldman et al., "A 24-week, randomized, double-blind study of donepezil in moderate to severe Alzheimer's disease," *Neurology*, 2001, 57: 613–620; B. Winblad et al., "A 1-year, randomized, placebo-controlled study of donepezil in mild to moderate AD," *Neurology*, 2001, 57: 489–495; P.N. Tariot et al., "A 5-month, randomized, placebo-controlled trial of galantamine in AD," *Neurology*, 2000, 54: 2269–2276.

29. C. Holmes et al., "The efficacy of donepezil in the treatment of neuro-psychiatric symptoms in Alzheimer disease," *Neurology*, 2004, 63: 214–219.

30. Barry Reisberg et al., "Memantine in moderate to severe Alzheimer's disease," *N Engl J Med*, 2003, 348: 1333–1341.

31. David Drachman, "Safe driving: Aging and Alzheimer's disease," *Neurology*, 2004, 63: 765.

32. Baoxi Qu et al., "Gene vaccination to bias the immune response to amyloid-beta peptide as therapy for Alzheimer disease," *Arch Neurol*, 2004, 61: 1859–1864; Shoji Tsuji, "DNA vaccination may open up a new avenue for treatment of Alzheimer disease," *Arch Neurol*, 2004, 61: 1832; A.J. Bayer et al., "Evaluation of the safety and immunogenicity of synthetic Abeta42 (AN1792) in patients with AD," *Neurology*, 2005, 64: 94–101; E. Masliah et al., "Abeta vaccination effects on plaque pathology in the absence of encephalitis in Alzheimer disease," *Neurology*, 2005, 64: 129–131.

33. S. Gilman et al., "Clinical effects of Abeta immunization (AN1792) in patients with AD in an interrupted trial," *Neurology*, 2005, 64: 1553–1662.

34. Margot O'Toole et al., "Risk factors associated with beta-amyloid 42 immunotherapy in preimmunization gene expression patterns of blood cells," *Arch Neurol*, 2005, 62: 1531–1536.

35. Charlene Laino, "In preliminary study, IVIG shows promise for Alzheimer's disease," *Neurology Today*, June 2005: 44–47.

36. Craig W. Ritchie et al., "Metal-protein attenuation with Iodochlorhydroxyquin (Clioquinal) targeting abeta amyloid deposition and toxicity in Alzheimer's disease," *Arch Neurol*, 2003, 60: 1685–1691.

37. Hiroaki Fukumoto et al., "Beta-secretase protein and activity are increased in the neocortex in Alzheimer's disease," *Arch Neurol*, 2002, 59: 1381–1389.

38. "Options for Alzheimer's continue to progress," *Neura Special Report*, Highlights of the 56th Annual Meeting of the AAN, April–May (2005).

39. Andrew Pollack, "In small trial, gene therapy is seen as aid in Alzheimer's," *New York Times*, April 25, 2005, C 9; Colby Strong, "Gene therapy slows progression of Alzheimer's disease," *Neurology Reviews*, June 2005 13, 6: 1, 69.

40. Jean McCann, "Intranasal insulin shows promise for Alzheimer's disease," *Neurology Reviews*, January 2005: 48–49.

CHAPTER 4: FRONTO-TEMPORAL DEMENTIA—PICK'S DISEASE

1. William Butler Yeats, "Two Songs from a Play," *The New Oxford Book of English Verse*, Oxford University Press, New York, 1984, Poem 772.

2. Rudolph Tanzi, "Tangles and neurodegenerative disease—A surprising twist," *N Engl J Med*, 2005, 353: 1853–1855.

3. S.A.R.B. Rombouts et al., "Loss of frontal fMRI activation in early frontotemporal dementia compared to early AD," *Neurology*, 2003, 60: 1904–1908.

4. W. Liu, "Behavioral disorders in the frontal and temporal variants of frontotemporal dementia," *Neurology*, 2004, 62: 742–748.

5. Ibid.

6. W.W. Seeley et al., "The natural history of temporal variant frontotemporal dementia," *Neurology*, 2005, 64: 1384–1390; Sian Thompson et al., "Left/right asymmetry of atrophy in semantic dementia," *Neurology*, 2003, 61: 1196–1203.

7. M. Marsel Mesulam, "Primary progressive aphasia—A language-based dementia," *N Engl J Med*, 2003, 349: 1535–1542.

8. Ibid.

9. Bruce Miller and Craig Hou, "Portraits of artists—Emergence of visual creativity in dementia," *Arch Neurol*, 2004, 61: 842–844.

CHAPTER 5: DEMENTIA WITH LEWY BODIES AND PARKINSON'S DISEASE DEMENTIA

1. Aristotle, "On The Soul," *The Basic Works of Aristotle*, Random House, New York, 1941, p. 548.

2. Lao-Tzu, *Te Tao Ching*, Translated by Robert Henricks, Ballantine Books, New York, 1989, p. 32.

3. Meeting Review, "Reconsidering diagnostic criteria for dementia with Lewy bodies," *Reviews In Neurological Diseases*, 2004, 1, #1: 31–34.

4. H. Ohtake et al., "Beta-synuclein gene alterations in dementia with Lewy bodies," *Neurology*, 2004, 63: 805–811.

5. Carol Lippa and Ian McKeith, "Dementia with Lewy bodies—Improving diagnostic criteria," *Neurology*, 2003, 60: 1571–1572; A.R. Merdes et al., "Influence of Alzheimer pathology on clinical diagnostic accuracy in dementia with Lewy bodies," *Neurology*, 2003, 60: 1586–1590.

6. Daniel Murman et al., "The impact of parkinsonism on costs of care in patients with AD and dementia with Lewy bodies," *Neurology*, 2003, 61: 944–949.

7. D.A. Cousins et al., "Atrophy of the putamen in dementia with Lewy bodies but not Alzheimer's disease," *Neurology*, 2003, 61: 1191–1195.

8. Tatsuo Shimomura et al., "Cognitive loss in dementia with Lewy bodies and Alzheimer disease," *Arch Neurol*, 1998, 55: 1547–1552.

9. M.L. Kraybill et al., "Cognitive differences in dementia patients with autopsy-verified AD, Lewy body pathology, or both," *Neurology*, 2005, 64: 2069–2073.

10. T.J. Ferman et al., "DLB fluctuations," *Neurology*, 2004, 62: 181–187.

11. "Reconsidering diagnostic criteria for dementia with Lewy bodies," *Reviews in Neurological Diseases*, 2004, 1: 31–34.

12. P. Thaisetthawatkul et al., "Autonomic dysfunction in dementia with Lewy bodies," *Neurology*, 2004, 62: 1804–1809.

13. Christopher Goetz, "Early iconography of Parkinson's disease," *Handbook of Parkinson's Disease*, 3rd Edition, 2003: 1–16.

14. Ali H. Rajput et al., "Epidemiology of parkinsonism," *Handbook of Parkinson's Disease* 3rd Edition, 2003: 17–42.

15. Ibid.

16. Elan Louis et al., "Functional correlates and prevalence of mild parkinsonian signs in a community population of older people," *Arch Neurol*, 2005, 62: 297–302.

17. Ed Susman, "Anxiety early in life: Could it lead to Parkinson's disease?" *Neurology Today*, June 2005: 49.

18. Zbigniew Wszolek and Matthew Farrer, "Genetics," *Handbook of Parkinsons's Disease*, 3rd Edition, 2003: 325–327.

19. Dennis W. Dickson, "Neuropathology of parkinsonism," *Handbook of Parkinson's Disease*, 3rd Edition, 2003: 203–219.

20. Kapil D. Seithi, "Differential diagnosis of parkinsonism," *Handbook of Parkinson's Disease*, 3rd Edition, 2003: 43–69.

21. Douglas Gelb et al., "Diagnostic criteria for Parkinson's disease," *Arch Neurol*, 1999, 56: 33–39.

22. Ibid.

23. C.W.C. Tam. "Temporal lobe atrophy on MRI in Parkinson's disease with dementia," *Neurology*, 2005, 64: 861–865.

24. Douglas Gelb et al., "Diagnostic criteria for Parkinson's disease," *Arch Neurol*, 1999, 56: 33–39; Kenneth Marek et al., "Neuroimaging in Parkinson's disease," *Handbook of Parkinson's Disease*, 3rd Edition, 2003: 179–202.

25. D. Aarsland et al., "Prevalence of dementia in Parkinson's disease," *Arch Neurol*, 2003, 60: 387–392.

26. Daniel Z. Press, "Parkinson's disease dementia—A first step," *N Engl J Med*, 2004, 351: 2547–2549.

27. J. Green et al., "Cognitive impairments in advanced PD without dementia," *Neurology*, 2002, 59: 1320–1324.

28. Richard B. Dewey Jr., "Nonmotor symptoms of Parkinson's disease," *Handbook of Parkinson's Disease*, 3rd Edition, 2003: 109–126.

29. Jeffrey L. Cummings, "Parkinson's disease dementia," *Medical Crossfire*, 2005, 6, #9: 22–30.

30. U.P. Mosimann et al., "Visual perception in Parkinson's disease dementia and dementia with Lewy bodies," *Neurology*, 2004, 63: 2091–2096.

31. Clifford W. Shults et al., "Effects of Coenzyme Q10 in early Parkinson's disease," *Arch Neurol*, 2002, 59: 1541–1550.

32. Murat Emre et al., "Rivastigmine for dementia associated with Parkinson's disease," *N Engl J Med*, 2004, 351: 2509–2518.

CHAPTER 6: VASCULAR DEMENTIA AND MIXED DEMENTIA

1. Michael de Montaigne, *Essays On Experience*, Translated by J.M. Cohen, Penguin Books, New York, 1958, p. 355.

2. Ozaki Hosai, *The Haiku Handbook*, William J. Higginson, McGraw Hill Paperbacks, New York, 1983, p. 31.

3. Kenneth M. Langa et al., "Mixed dementia," *JAMA*, 2004, 292: 2901–2908.

4. O.L. Lopez et al., "Classification of vascular dementia in the cardiovascular health cognition study," *Neurology*, 2005, 64: 1539–1547.

5. L.H. Kuller et al., "Determinants of vascular dementia in the cardiovascular health cognition study," *Neurology*, 2005, 64: 1548–1552.

6. Tarja Pohjasvaara et al., "Dementia three months after stroke," *Stroke*, 1997, 28: 785–792.

7. J.S. Elkins et al., "Stroke risk factors and loss of high cognitive function," *Neurology*, 2004, 63: 793–799.

8. J.T. Moroney, "Risk factors for incident dementia after stroke," *Stroke*, 1996, 27: 1283–1289.

9. Natalie Phillips and C. Charles Mate-Kole, "Cognitive deficits in peripheral vascular disease," *Stroke*, 1997, 28: 777–784.

10. Gustavo Roman, "New insight into Binswanger's disease," *Arch Neurol*, 1999, 56: 1061–1062.

11. H.C. Chui et al., "Clinical criteria for the diagnosis of vascular dementia," *Arch Neurol*, 2000, 57: 191–196.

12. D. Wilkinson et al., "Donepezil in vascular dementia," *Neurology*, 2003, 61: 479–486; T. Erkinjuntti et al., "Efficacy of galantamine in probable vascular dementia and Alzheimer's disease combined with cerebrovascular disease," *Lancet*, 2002, 359: 1283–1290.

CHAPTER 7: LESS COMMON FORMS OF DEMENTIA

1. May Sarton, *Kinds of Love*, W.W. Norton & Company, New York, 1994, p. 115.

2. R.D. Adams et al., "Symptomatic occult hydrocephalus with 'normal' cerebrospinal fluid pressure," *N Engl J Med*, 1965, 273: 117–126.

3. Markus Glatzel et al., "Human prion diseases," *Arch Neurol*, 2005, 62: 545–562.

4. "Classic CJD," *Homepage CDC*; accessed on 7/21/05 at www.cdc.gov/nicidod/dvrd/cjd/1–2

5. Herbert R. Karp and Suzanne Mirra, "Dementia in adults," *Clinical Neurology, Baker and Baker*, 1976, Volume 2, Chapter 32: 41–45.

6. T. Hamaguchi et al., "Clinical diagnosis of MM2-type sporadic Creutzfeldt-Jakob disease," *Neurology*, 2005, 64: 643–648.

7. Martin Zeidler and Alison Green, "Advances in diagnosis of Creutzfeldt-Jakob disease with MRI and CSF 14-3-3 protein analysis," *Neurology*, 2004, 63: 410–411.

8. B. Meissner et al., "Sporadic Creutzfeldt-Jakob disease—Magnetic resonance imaging and clinical findings," *Neurology*, 2004, 63: 450–456.

9. R.G. Will et al., "A new variant of Creutzfeldt-Jakob disease in the UK," *Lancet*, 1996, 347: 921–925.

10. "Fact Sheet: New variant Creutzfeldt-Jakob disease," *CDC Web Page*; accessed on 1/20/04 www.cdc.gov/nicidod/dvrd/vcjd/

11. Y. Tsuboi et al., "Atrophy of superior cerebellar peduncle in progressive supranuclear palsy," *Neurology*, 2003, 60: 1766–1769; H. Oba et al., "New and reliable MRI diagnosis for progressive supranuclear palsy," *Neurology*, 2005, 64: 2050–2055.

12. Fletcher McDowell and Jesse Cedarbaum, "The extrapyramidal system and disorders of movement," *Clinical Neurology Baker and Baker*, 1987, Volume 3, Chapter 38: 49–57.

13. E.H. Aylard et al., "Onset and rate of striatal atrophy in preclinical Huntington's disease," *Neurology*, 2004, 63: 66–72.

14. "Alzheimer's drug holds promise in Huntington's disease," *Neura*, highlights of the 56th Annual Meeting of the American Academy of Neurology, April 24–May 1, 2004, p. 9.

CHAPTER 8: ACCELERATED AGING, COGNITIVE RESERVE AND WHAT WE CAN'T CONTROL

1. Ashley Montagu, *Growing Young*, McGraw Hill, New York, 1981, p. 3.

2. Priest Saigyo, *The Penguin Book of Japanese Verse*, Translated by Geoffrey Bownas and Anthony Thwaite, New York, 1983, p. 101.

3. J. Luchsinger et al., "Aggregation of vascular risk factors and risk of incident Alzheimer disease," *Neurology*, 2005, 65: 545–551.

4. B.M. Van Gelder et al., "Physical activity in relation to cognitive decline in elderly men," *Neurology*, 2004, 63: 2316–2321.

5. Jennifer Weuve et al., "Physical activity, including walking, and cognitive function in older women," *JAMA*, 2004, 292: 1454–1461; Robert Abbott, et al., "Walking and dementia in physically capable elderly men," *JAMA*, 2004, 292: 1447–1453.

6. Jose Luchsinger et al, "Caloric intake and the risk of Alzheimer disease," *Arch Neurol*, 2002, 59: 1258–1263.

7. Cristina Geroldi et al., "Insulin resistance in cognitive impairment," *Arch Neurol*, 2005, 62: 1067–1072.

8. Iris Goldstein et al., "Ambulatory blood pressure and the brain," *Neurology*, 2005, 64: 1846–1852.

9. A. Ott et al., "Smoking and risk of dementia and Alzheimer's disease in a population-based cohort study: The Rotterdam study," *Lancet*, 1998, 351: 1840–1843; J. Luchsinger et al., "Aggregation of vascular risk factors and risk of incident Alzheimer disease," *Neurology*, 2005, 65: 545–561.

10. A. Ott et al., "Effect of smoking on global cognitive function in nondemented elderly," *Neurology*, 2004, 62: 920–924.

11. R. Brunner et al., "Effect of corticosteroids on short-term and long-term memory," *Neurology*, 2005, 64: 335–337.

12. Robert Green et al., "Depression as a risk factor for Alzheimer disease," *Arch Neurol*, 2003, 60: 753–759.

13. M.F. Newman et al., "Longitudinal assessment of neurocognitive function after coronary artery bypass surgery," *N Engl J Med*, 2001, 344: 395–402.

14. Ola Selnes and Guy McKhann, "Late cognitive decline after CABG," *Neurology*, 2002, 59: 660–661.

15. Jae Kang et al., "Postmenopausal hormone therapy and risk of cognitive decline in community dwelling aging women," *Neurology*, 2004, 63: 101–107.

16. M. Muller et al., "Endogenous sex hormone levels and cognitive function in aging men," *Neurology*, 2005, 64: 866–871.

17. Nikolaos Scarmeas et al., "Association of life activities with cerebral blood flow in Alzheimer disease," *Arch Neurol*, 2003, 60: 359–365.

CHAPTER 9: THE IMPORTANCE OF PHYSICAL ACTIVITY AND EXERCISE

1. James Churchill et al., "Exercise, experience and the aging brain," *Neurobiology of Ageing*, 2002, 23: 941–955.

2. Arthur Kramer et al., "Aging, fitness and neurocognitive function," *Nature*, 1999, 400: 418–419.

3. Danielle Laurin et al., "Physical activity and risk of cognitive impairment and dementia in elderly persons," *Arch Neurol*, 2001, 58: 498–504; Robert Abbott et al., "Walking and dementia in physically capable elderly men," *JAMA*, 2004, 292: 1447–1453; Jennefer Weuve et al., "Physical activity, including walking, and cognitive function in older women," *JAMA*, 2004, 292: 1454–1461; B.M. Van Gelder et al., "Physical activity in relation to cognitive decline in elderly men," *Neurology*, 2004, 63: 2316–2321.

4. Carl Cotman and Nichole Berchtold, "Exercise: A behavioral intervention to enhance brain health and plasticity," *Trends in Neurosciences*, 2002, 25: 295–301.

5. Laurin et al., "Physical activity," *Arch Neurol*. See note 3.

6. Weuve et al., "Cognitive function in older women," *JAMA*. See note 3.

7. Abbott et al., "Walking and dementia," *JAMA*. See note 3.

8. Suvi Rovio et al., "Leisure-time physical activity at midlife and the risk of dementia and Alzheimer's disease," *Lancet Neurol*, 2005, 4: 705–711.

9. H. Chen et al., "Physical activity and the risk of Parkinson's disease," *Neurology*, 2005, 64: 664–669.

10. Morimasa Kato et al., "Differential physical activity between MCI and normal elderly people—Tone project," *Alzheimer's and Dementia*, 2005, 1: S63.

11. James Churchill et al., "Exercise, experience and aging brain," *Neurobiology of Aging*. See note 1.

12. Chong Do Lee et al., "Physical activity and stroke risk," *Stroke*, 2003, 34: 2475–2482.

13. Abbott et al., "Walking and dementia," *JAMA*. See note 3.

14. C. Justin Romano, "Modifiable risk factors for Alzheimer's disease," *Neurology Reviews*, September 2004, Volume 12, #9: 1, 54, 56.

15. James Churchill et al., "Exercise, experience, and aging brain," *Neurobiology of Aging*. See note 1.

16. Carl Cotman and Nicole Berchtold, "Exercise," *Trends in Neurosciences*. See note 4.

17. Ibid.

18. James Churchill et al., "Exercise, experience and aging brain," *Neurobiology of Aging*. See note 1.

19. Carl Cotman and Nicole Berchtold, "Exercise," *Trends in Neurosciences*. See note 4.

20. Carl Cotman and Nicole Berchtold, "Exercise," *Trends in Neurosciences*. See note 4.

21. C. Justin Romano, "Risk factors for Alzheimer's disease," *Neurology Reviews*. See note 14.

22. Jane Brody, "Panel urges hour of exercise a day; Sets diet guidelines," *New York Times*, September 6, 2002.

23. Hideaki Soya et al., "Enhanced memory function of elderly people by exercise intervention with enjoyable and mild intensity: Tone project," *Alzheimer's and Dementia*, 2005, 1: S98.

24. Elizabeth Weil, "Fitness can be a work in progress," *New York Times*, September 27, 2005, p. G10.

CHAPTER 10: THE NEED FOR COGNITIVE STIMULATION AND SOCIALIZATION

1. Aristotle, "Metaphysics," *The Basic Works of Aristotle*, Random House, New York, 1941, p. 689.

2. Henry Ford, quoted in Helen Nearing, *Light on Aging and Dying*, Tilbury House Publishers, Gardiner, Maine, 1995, p. 4.

3. N.W. Milgram et al., "Learning ability in aged beagle dogs is preserved by behavioral enrichment and dietary fortification: A two year longitudinal study," *Neurobiology of Aging*, 2005, 26: 77–90.

4. Joanna Jankowsky et al., "Environmental enrichment mitigates cognitive deficits in APP/PSI transgenic mice," *Alzheimer's and Dementia*, 2005, 1: S99.

5. Robert Wilson et al., "Participation in cognitively stimulating activities and risk of incident Alzheimer disease," *JAMA*, 2002, 287: 742–748; Joe Verghese et al., "Leisure activities and the risk of dementia in the elderly," *N Engl J Med*, 2003, 348: 2508–2516; R.S. Wilson et al., "Cognitive activity and incident AD in a population-based sample of older persons," *Neurology*, 2002, 59: 1910–1914; N. Scarmeas et al., "Influence of leisure activity on the incidence of Alzheimer's disease," *Neurology*, 2001, 57: 2236–2242.

6. Robert Wilson et al., "Participation in cognitively stimulating activities," *JAMA*. See note 5.

7. Joe Verghese et al., "Leisure activities," *N Engl J Med*. See note 5.

8. Robert Wilson et al., "Cognitive activity," *Neurology*. See note 5.

9. N. Scarmeas et al., "Influence of leisure activity," *Neurology*. See note 5.

10. Carl Cotman and Nicole Berchtold, "Exercise: A behavioral intervention to enhance brain health and plasticity," *Trends in Neurosciences*, 2002, 25: 295–301.

11. Ibid.

12. James Churchill et al., "Exercise, experience and the aging brain," *Neurobiology of Aging*, 2002, 23: 941–955.

13. Sara Rimer, "An Alaska trek makes elders of the aging," *New York Times*, September 2, 1998.

14. Karlene Ball et al., "Effects of cognitive training interventions with older adults," *JAMA*, 2002, 288: 2271–2281.

15. J. Olazaran et al., "Benefits of cognitive-motor intervention in MCI and mild to moderate Alzheimer disease," *Neurology*, 2004, 63: 2348–2353.

CHAPTER 11: DIET AND SUBSTANCES THAT MAY REDUCE THE RISK OF DEMENTIA

1. Robert Friedland, "Fish consumption and the risk of Alzheimer disease," *Arch Neurol*, 2003, 60: 923–924.

2. Martha Clare Morris et al., "Consumption of fish and omega-3 fatty acids and risk of incident Alzheimer disease," *Arch Neurol*, 2003, 60: 940–946.

3. S. Kalmijn, "Fatty acid intake and the risk of dementia and cognitive decline: A review of clinical and epidemiological studies," *J Nutr Health Aging*, 2000, 4: 194.

4. M.J. Ebgelhart et al., "Diet and risk of dementia: Does fat matter?" *Neurology*, 2002, 59: 1915–1921.

5. F. Tchantchou et al., "Dietary supplementation with apple juice concentrate alleviates the compensatory increase in glutathione synthase transcription and activity that accompanies dietary and genetically-induced oxidative stress," *The Journal of Nutrition, Health and Aging*, 2004: 1–5.

6. Amy Borenstein et al., "Consumption of fruit and vegetable juices predicts a reduced risk of Alzheimer's disease: The Kame project," *Alzheimer's and Dementia*, 2005, 1, Suppl 1 S60

7. Kavon Rezai-Zedah et al., "Green tea epigallocatechin-3-gallate (EGCG) modulates amyloid precursor protein cleavage and reduces cerebral amyloidosis in Alzheimer transgenic mice," *J Neurosci*, 2005, 25: 8807–8814.

8. Linda Carroll, "NSAIDS—once deemed promising—Suspended in Alzheimer trial," *Neurology Today*, February 2005: 40–52.

9. B.A. In't Veld et al., "Nonsteroidal anti-inflammatory drugs and the risk of Alzheimer's disease," *N Engl J Med*, 2001, 345: 1515–1521.

10. Peter Zandi, "Reduced incidence of AD with NSAID but not H2 receptor antagonists," *Neurology*, 2002, 59: 880–886.

11. Linda Carroll, "NSAIDS," *Neurology Today*. See note 8.

12. Larry Schuster, "Ibuprofen, but not other NSAIDs protects against Parkinson's disease," *Neurology Today*, June 2005: 47.

13. Victor Sierpina, Berndt Wollschlaeger, Mark Blumenthal, "Ginko biloba," *Am Fam Phys*, 2003, 68: 923–926.

14. G. Li et al., "Statin therapy and risk of dementia in the elderly," *Neurology*, 2004, 63: 1624–1628.

15. C. Dufouil et al., "APOE genotype, cholesterol level, lipid-lowering treatment and dementia," *Neurology*, 2005, 64: 1531–1538.

16. Kathleen Hayden et al., "Statin use does not reduce cognitive decline in the elderly. The Cache County study," *Alzheimer's and Dementia*, 2005, 1: S97.

17. L.R. Wagstaff et al., "Statin-associated memory loss: Analysis of 60 case reports and review of the literature," *Pharmacotherapy*, 2003, 7: 871–80.

18. M. Sano et al., "A controlled trial of selegiline, alpha-tocopherol, or both as treatment for Alzheimer's disease," *N Engl J Med*, 1997, 336: 1216–1222.

19. M. C. Morris et al., "Vitamin E and cognitive decline in older persons," *Arch Neurol*, 2002, 59: 1125–1132.

20. P.P. Zandi et al., "Reduced risk of Alzheimer's disease in users of antioxidant vitamin supplements: The Cache County study," *Arch Neurol*, 2004, 61: 82–88.

21. Deborah Blacker, "Mild cognitive impairment—No benefit from vitamin E, little from donepezil," *N Engl J Med*, 2005, 352: 2439–2441.

22. Ronald Peterson et al., "Vitamin E and donepezil for the treatment of mild cognitive impairment," *N Engl J Med*, 2005, 352: 2379–2388.

23. S.M. Zhang et al., "Intakes of vitamins E and C, carotenoids, vitamin supplements, and PD risk," *Neurology*, 2002, 59: 1161–1169.

24. Martha Clare Morris et al., "Relation of the tocopherol forms to incident Alzheimer disease and to cognitive change," *Am J Clin Nutr*, 2005, 81: 508–514.

25. Sudha Seshadri et al., "Plasma homocysteine as a risk factor for dementia and Alzheimer's disease," *N Engl J Med*, 2002, 346: 476–483.

26. J.W. Miller et al., "Homocysteine, vitamin B6, and vascular disease in Alzheimer's patients," *Neurology*, 2002, 58: 1471–1475.

27. James Toole and Clifford Jack, "Food (and vitamins) for thought," *Neurology*, 2002, 58: 1449–1450.

28. H-X. Wang et al., "Vitamin B12 and folate in relation to the development of Alzheimer's disease," *Neurology*, 2001, 56: 1188–1194.

29. M.C. Morris et al., "Dietary niacin and the risk of incident Alzheimer's disease and of cognitive decline," *J Neurol Neurosurg Psychiatry*, 2004, 75: 1093–1099.

30. C.W. Shults, "Effects of Coenzyme Q10 in early Parkinson's disease: Evidence of slowing of the functional decline," *Arch Neurol*, 2002, 59: 10.

31. C.W. Shults and A. Schapira, "A cue to queue for CoQ?" *Neurology*, 2001, 57: 375–376.

32. F. De Bustos et al., "Serum levels of Coenzyme Q10 in patients with Alzheimer's disease," *Journal of Neural Transmission*, 2000, 107: 233–239.

33. F. Yang et al., "Curcumin inhibits formation of amyloid beta oligomers and fibrils and binds plaques and reduces amyloid in vivo," *J. Biol. Chem*; accessed at www.jbc.org/cgi/content/abstract/M404751200V1 on December 7, 2004.

34. Meir Stampfer et al., "Effects of moderate alcohol consumption on cognitive function in women," *N Engl J Med*, 2005, 352: 245–253.

35. Thomas Truelsen et al., "Amount and type of alcohol and risk of dementia," *Neurology*, 2002, 59: 1313–1319.

36. T. Ohrui et al., "Effects of brain-penetrating ACE inhibitors on Alzheimer's disease progression," *Neurology*, 2004, 63: 1324.

37. S.D. Moffat et al., "Free testosterone and risk for Alzheimer disease in older men," *Neurology*, 2004, 62: 188–193.

38. Victor Henderson and Eva Hogervorst, "Testosterone and Alzheimer disease," *Neurology*, 2004, 62: 170–171.

39. M.M. Cherrier et al., "Testosterone supplementation improves spatial and verbal memory in healthy older men," *Neurology*, 2001, 57: 80–88.

40. Sally Shumaker et al., "Estrogen plus progestin and the incidence of dementia and mild cognitive impairment in postmenopausal women," *JAMA*, 2003, 289: 2651–2662; Sally Shumaker et al., "Conjugated equine estrogens and incidence of probable dementia and mild cognitive impairment in post menopausal women," *JAMA*, 2004, 291: 2947–2958.

41. S. Gillette-Guyonnet et al., "Cognitive impairment and composition of drinking water in women," *Am J Clin Nutr*, 2005, 81: 897–902.

42. Monisha Sharma et al., "Protective effect of alpha lipoic acid and trans resveratrol on spatial memory deficits caused by intracerebroventricular streptozotocin in rats," *Alzheimer's and Dementia*, 2005, 1: S69.

AFTERWORD

1. Lao-Tzu, *Te Tao Ching*, Translated by Robert Henricks, Ballantine Books, New York, 1989, p. 85.

GLOSSARY

acetylcholine: an important neurotransmitter, critical for memory.

agnosia: an impairment of the ability to recognize.

Alzheimer's disease: a neurodegenerative disease that causes dementia.

amyloid: a complex protein that is greatly increased in the brain in Alzheimer's disease.

aphasia: an impairment of language with an inability to speak, or understand speech.

APOE (Apolipoprotein E): a protein involved in cholesterol transport. There are three genetically determined forms. An increased risk of Alzheimer's is seen with the APOE 4 form.

apraxia: an impairment in the performance of skilled or purposeful movements while motor ability and comprehension remain intact.

atherosclerosis: fatty deposits and plaques in the lining of the arteries that can obstruct blood flow and lead to clots.

axon: the major process of a neuron that conducts impulses away from the cell body.

cerebral: relating to the hemispheres of the brain.

cerebral cortex: the cellular mantle covering the surface of the hemispheres of the brain.

cholinesterase: enzymes that break down the neurotransmitter acetylcholine.

clinical: relating to the symptoms and course of a disease.

CT scan (Computed Tomography Scan): a series of x-rays through a section of the body that can be reconstructed by a computer into images in different planes for interpretation.

demographics: the study of populations, their characteristics and statistics.

dendrites: the smaller branching processes of the neurons.

disinhibition: loss of social restraint; often associated with frontal lobe dysfunction.

dopamine: an important neurotransmitter involved in emotions and motor activity.

enzymes: proteins that act as catalysts necessary for certain chemical reactions.

fMRI (Functional Magnetic Resonance Imaging): an MRI technique that can spotlight areas of brain activity induced by thought or action.

free radicals: compounds that are unstable chemically, existing transiently in an uncombined state. In the brain, these can damage and destroy neurons.

fronto-temporal dementia: a neurodegenerative disease that causes dementia.

hippocampus: a body of cells deep in the temporal lobes essential for memory.

hypoxic, or hypoxia: diminished oxygen supply.

ischemia or ischemic: diminished blood supply usually because of narrowing or blockage of an artery.

Lewy body disease: a neurodegenerative disease that causes dementia.

metabolic, metabolism: the sum of chemical and physical activities in cells and tissues.

MRI scan (Magnetic Resonance Imaging): similar to CT scan but performed with magnetic waves instead of radiation.

myelin: fatty substance around nerve fibers that permits better conduction of electrical impulses.

neurons (nerve cells): the brain cells responsible for thinking, movement and perception of sensation.

neurotransmitters: the chemicals that transmit impulses across the gap between neurons.

oxidation: a reaction that combines oxygen with another substance and may release free radicals as a byproduct.

oxidative stress: injury to brain cells because of oxidation and free radicals.

pathological, pathology: relating to the nature, causes, and structural changes resulting from disease.

PET scan (Positron Emission Tomography): a computerized scan done with radioactive isotopes that concentrate in particular cells. When done with glucose, it tracks active metabolism.

SPECT scan (Single Photon Emission Computed Tomography): computerized imaging with radioactive isotopes that shows metabolic and physiologic functions of tissues.

synapse: the connection between two neurons including a gap between the cells transversed by neurotransmitters.

tau protein: a protein associated with, and stabilizing the microtubules of the cell. When hyperphosphorylated (a chemical reaction involving phosphorous) in Alzheimer's disease, it forms neurofibrillary tangles. It also plays a role in diseases called tauopathies.

vascular: relating to the blood vessels, particularly the arteries.

INDEX

About the Author

ROBERT LEVINE, M.D., is former Chief of Neurology at Norwalk Hospital and retired Associate Clinical Professor of Medicine at Yale University School of Medicine.